ABC OF EYES
Second edition

To our parents

ABC OF EYES

SECOND EDITION

P T KHAW MRCP FRCS FRCOphth
Consultant ophthalmic surgeon
Moorfields Eye Hospital, London

and

A R ELKINGTON FRCS FRCOphth
Professor of ophthalmology
University of Southampton
President, Royal College of Ophthalmologists

BMJ
Publishing
Group

First published in 1988
by the BMJ Publishing Group, BMA House, Tavistock Square,
London WC1H 9JR

First published 1988
Second impression 1990
Third impression 1991
Fourth impression 1992
Fifth impression 1992
Sixth impression 1992
Seventh impression 1993
Eighth impression 1993
Second edition 1994

British Library Cataloguing in Publication Data

A catalogue record for this book is available
from the British Library

ISBN 0-7279-0766-2

Printed in Singapore, by Craft Print Pte Ltd.
Typesetting by Apek Typesetters, Nailsea, Bristol, Avon

Contents

ACKNOWLEDGMENTS

We acknowledge the help and feedback we have received over the years from medical students, general practitioners, ophthalmologists, optometrists, and orthoptists at Southampton University and Moorfields Eye Hospital. We would like to thank Peggy Khaw for her work and support with both editions, Peter Jack and Humera Shad for drawing the diagrams and Humera Shad and Vicki Scott for their help with the second edition. Christine Astin has been very helpful with the chapter on refractive errors. Jane Smith, Mary Evans, Mary Banks and Deborah Reece have also been tremendously supportive, steering us through the pitfalls of publishing. We also thank David Gartry and Linda Ficker for their advice on the refractive surgery section. Jackie Howe and Maggie Parker of the Royal London Society for the Blind/Moorfields Eye Hospital support service for the visually disabled have given us the benefit of their tremendous experience in the section on services for the visually handicapped. Finally, we would like to thank the Guide Dogs for the Blind Association for permission to reproduce their photograph of a guide dog on page 41, and Pharmacia for permission to use three of their colour plates of cataract surgery on page 27.

P T K
A R E

HISTORY AND EXAMINATION

History

As in all clinical medicine, an accurate history and examination are essential if the correct diagnosis and treatment are to be achieved. Most ocular conditions can be diagnosed with a good history and simple examination techniques. Conversely, failure to take a history and do a simple examination may lead to loss of sight or even life threatening conditions being missed.

The history may give clues to the diagnosis. Important points in the ophthalmic history obviously include visual symptoms.

The rate of onset of visual symptoms gives an indication of the cause. A rapid deterioration in vision tends to be vascular in origin, whereas a gradual onset suggests a cause such as cataract. The loss of visual field may be characteristic, such as the central field loss of macular degeneration. Symptoms such as flashing lights may indicate traction on the retina and impending retinal detachment.

It is particularly important to assess the effect of the visual disability on lifestyle, and difficulties with work, reading, watching television, and managing in the house should be identified. This is important in assessing the impact of the visual disability on the patient, especially when a condition such as cataract can now be operated on at an early stage with modern techniques.

The patient should also be asked exactly what worries him as visual symptoms often cause great anxiety. Appropriate reassurance can then be given.

> **Visual symptoms**
>
> - Monocular or binocular
> - Type of disturbance
> - Rate of onset
> - Presence and type of field loss
> - Associated symptoms—for example, flashing lights, floaters
> - Effect on lifestyle

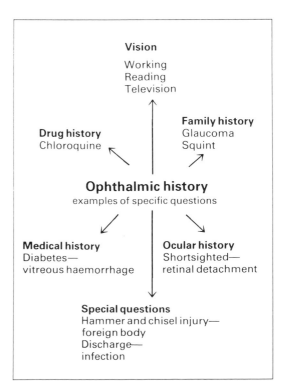

Questions about the particular symptom

Some specific questions are important in certain circumstances. If there has been ocular trauma, a history of any high velocity injury—particularly a hammer and chisel injury—should suggest an intraocular foreign body. Other questions—for example, about the type of discharge—may allow the diagnosis to be made in a patient with a red eye.

Ocular history is easily forgotten but is essential. The patient's red eye may be associated with contact lens wear. A history of severe shortsightedness (myopia) considerably increases the risk of retinal detachment. Patients often forget to mention eye drops and eye operations if they are just asked about "drugs and operations."

Medical history—Many systemic disorders affect the eye, and the medical history may give clues to the cause of the problem—for instance, a vitreous haemorrhage in a patient with diabetes.

Family history—The best example of the importance of the family history is in the case of chronic open angle glaucoma. This may be asymptomatic until severe visual damage has occurred. The risk of the disease is 1:10 in first degree relatives, and the disease may be arrested at an early stage. A family history of squint is also a risk factor in the development of squint.

Drug history—Many drugs affect the eyes, and they should always be considered as a cause of ocular problems—for example, chloroquine may affect the retina.

Examination of the visual system

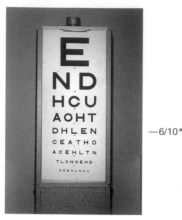

—6/10*

*Approximate level on Snellen chart required in at least one eye for driving a car.

Assessment of vision

- Snellen chart at 6 metres
- Snellen chart closer
- Counting fingers
- Hand movements
- Perception of light
- No perception of light

Testing visual fields.

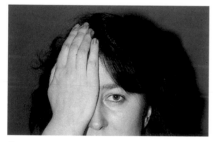

Ask patient to cover eye not being tested. Ensure that eye is completely covered by palm.

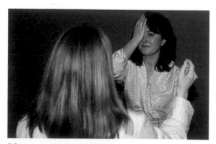

Move red pin in from periphery and ask patient to say when it is visible.

Vision

An assessment of visual acuity is fundamental in any ocular disorder as it measures the function of the eye and gives some idea of the patient's disability. It may also have considerable medicolegal implications, as in the case of ocular damage at work or after assault.

Visual acuity is checked using a standard Snellen chart at six metres. If there is no room large enough a mirror can be used with a reversed Snellen chart at three metres. The numbers under the letters indicate the distance at which a person with no refractive error can read that line (hence the 6/60 line should normally be read at 60 metres). If the top line cannot be discerned the test can be done closer to the chart. If the chart cannot be read at one metre patients may be asked to count fingers, and, if they cannot do that, to detect hand movements. Finally, it may be that they can perceive only light. From the patients' point of view the functional difference between these categories may be the difference between managing at home on their own (counting fingers) and total dependence on others (perception of light).

Vision should be tested with the aid of the patient's usual glasses or contact lenses. To achieve the optimal visual acuity the patient should be asked to look through a pin hole. This reduces the effect of any refractive error. It is particularly useful if the patient cannot use contact lenses because of a red eye or has not brought his glasses. If patients cannot read English they can be asked to match letters; this is also useful for young children.

Reading vision can be tested using a standard reading type book or, if this is not available, various sizes of newpaper print. There may be quite a difference in the near and distance vision. A good example is presbyopia, which usually develops in the late 40s owing to the failure of accommodation with age. Distance vision may be 6/6 without glasses but the patient may be able to read only larger newspaper print.

Field of vision

Testing the visual field may give clues to the site of any lesion and the diagnosis.

Location of the lesion—Unilateral field loss in the lower nasal field suggests an upper temporal retinal lesion. Central field loss usually indicates macular problems. A homonymous hemianopia indicates problems in the brain rather than the eye, though the patient may present with visual disturbance.

Diagnosis—If the patient has a bitemporal field defect this is most commonly due to a pituitary tumour. A field defect arching over central vision to the blind spot (arcuate scotoma) is almost pathognomonic of glaucoma.

To test the visual field—The patient should be seated directly opposite the examiner and should then be asked to cover the eye that is not being tested and to look at the examiner's face. If there is a gross defect the patient will not be able to see part of the examiner's face and may be able to indicate this precisely: "I can't see the centre of your face."

If no gross defect is present the fields can be tested more formally. Testing the visual field using finger movements peripherally will show severe defects, but a more sensitive test is the detection of red colour, because the ability to detect red tends to be affected earlier. A red pin is moved in from the periphery and the patient is asked when he can see something red. Finally, an extremely sensitive test is the comparison of the red in different quadrants. A good example is a patient who may have clinical signs of pituitary disease such as acromegaly; an early temporal defect can be detected if the patient is asked to compare the "quality" of the red in the upper temporal and nasal fields.

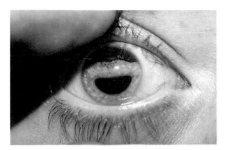

Torn peripheral iris (iridodialysis).

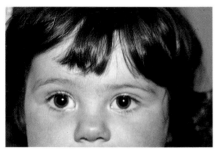

Distorted pupil after broad iridectomy.

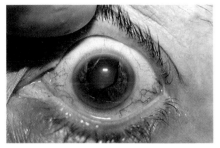

Normal position of corneal light reflexes.

The pupils

Careful inspection of the pupils can show signs that are helpful in diagnosis. A bright torch is essential. A pupil stuck down to the lens is due to inflammation within the eye, which is always serious. A peaked pupil after ocular injury suggests perforation with iris trapped in the wound. **Abnormal pupil reactions in the presence of ocular symptoms should always be treated seriously.**

The pupils' reactions to light are a simple way of checking the integrity of the visual pathways. By the time the pupils do not react to direct light, however, the damage is extremely severe. A much more sensitive test is the relative difference in pupillary reactions. A bright torch light is moved to and fro between the eyes not allowing time for the pupils to dilate. If one of the pupils does dilate when the light shines on it, there is a defect in the visual pathway on that side. Cataracts and macular degeneration do not usually cause an afferent pupillary defect unless the lesions are particularly advanced. Neurological disease must be suspected.

Other important and potentially life threatening conditions in which the pupils are affected include Horner's syndrome, where the pupil is small but reactive and there is associated ptosis. This condition may be caused by an apical lung carcinoma. The well known Argyll Robertson pupils caused by syphilis are rare. In a third nerve palsy the pupil is dilated and usually accompanied by ptosis; in this case the eye is divergent. Causes include a treatable intracranial aneurysm.

Eye position and movements

The appearance of the eyes will show the presence of any large degree of misalignment. This can, however, be misleading if the medial folds of the eyelid are wide. The position of the corneal reflections will help to confirm whether there is a true "squint". Squint and cover tests will be dealt with in the chapter on squint.

Patients should be asked if they have any double vision. If so, they should be asked to say whether diplopia occurs in any particular direction of gaze. It is important to exclude third (eye turned out) or sixth (failure of abduction) nerve palsies as these may be secondary to life threatening conditions. Complex abnormalities of eye movements should lead one to suspect myasthenia gravis or dysthyroid eye disease.

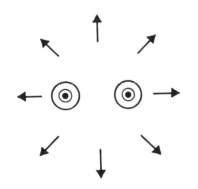

Eye movements.

- Test movements in all directions and also convergence
- Ask about double vision: if present, in which direction of gaze is it most pronounced?
- Look for nystagmus

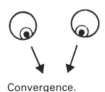

Convergence.

Eyelids: compare both sides and note position, lid lesions, and conditions of margins.

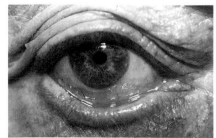

Ectropion.

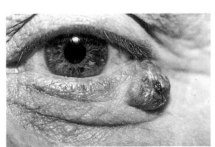

Basal cell carcinoma.

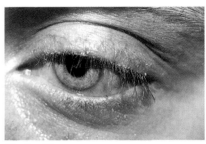

Blepharitis.

History and examination

Conjunctiva and sclera:
- Look for local or generalised inflammation
- Pull down lower lid and evert upper lid

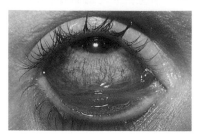

Conjunctivitis.

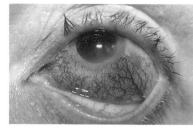

Scleritis.

Cornea:
- Look at clarity
- Stain with fluorescein

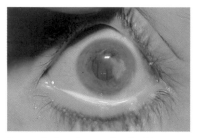

Corneal abrasion stained with fluorescein and illuminated with blue light.

Anterior chamber:
- Check for blood and pus
- Check chamber depth

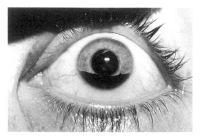

Blood in anterior chamber (hyphaema).

The following pieces of equipment are required:
- A bright torch (with a blue filter for use with fluorescein)
- A magnifying aid
- Fluorescein impregnated strips or eye drops.

Examination of the eyelids, conjunctiva, sclera, and cornea should be performed in a good light and with magnification. The lower lid should be pulled down to show the conjunctival lining and any secretions that may be in the lower fornix. **The cornea should then be stained with fluorescein eye drops; if this is not done many lesions, including large corneal ulcers, may be missed.** The anterior chamber should be examined looking specifically at the depth and for the presence of pus or blood.

If there are symptoms of "grittiness," a red eye, or any history of foreign body the upper eyelid should be everted. This should not be done, however, if there is any question of ocular perforation as the ocular contents may prolapse.

Intraocular pressure

The assessment of intraocular pressure by palpation is useful only when the intraocular pressure is considerably raised, as in acute closed angle glaucoma. The closed eye should be gently palpated between two fingers and compared with the other eye or with the examiner's own eye. The eye with acute glaucoma feels hard. Acute angle closure should be considered in any person over the age of 50 with a red eye.

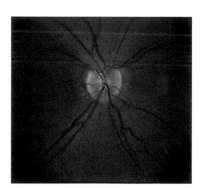

Normal disc.

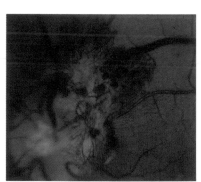

New vessels on optic disc in diabetes.

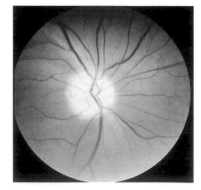

Optic atrophy.

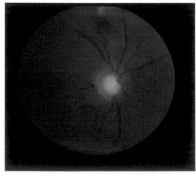

Glaucomatous cupping.

Ophthalmoscopy

Good ophthalmoscopy is essential if many serious ocular and general diseases are not to be missed. To get a good view the pupil should be dilated. There is a risk of precipitating acute angle closure glaucoma, but this is very small. Patients should be warned to seek help immediately if they have symptoms of pain or haloes around lights after having their pupils dilated. The best dilating drop is tropicamide 1%, which is short acting and has little effect on accommodation. The effects may, however, still last several hours and the patient should be warned not to drive until any blurring of vision has subsided.

The ophthalmoscope should be set on the 0 lens. Patients should be asked to fix their gaze on an object in the distance as this reduces pupillary constriction and keeps the eye still. To enable a patient to fix on a distant object with the other eye the examiner should use his right eye to examine the patient's right eye, and vice versa. The light should be shone at the eye until the red reflex is elicited. This red reflex is the reflection from the fundus. If this is absent or diminished there is an opacity between the cornea and the retina. The commonest opacity is a cataract.

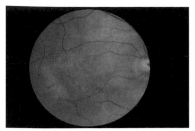

Age related macular degeneration.

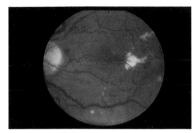

Diabetic maculopathy.

The optic disc should then be located and brought into focus with the lenses in the ophthalmoscope. If patients have large refractive errors they can be asked to leave their glasses on, though this can cause more reflections. The physical signs at the disc may be the only chance of detecting serious disease in the patient. A blurred disc edge may be the only sign of a cerebral tumour. Cupping of the optic disc may be the only sign of undetected primary open angle glaucoma. New vessels at the disc may herald blinding proliferative retinopathy in a patient without symptoms. A pale disc may be the only stigma of past attacks of optic neuritis, or of a compressive cerebral tumour.

The retina should be scanned for abnormalities such as haemorrhages, exudates, or new vessels. The green filter on the ophthalmoscope helps to enhance blood vessels and microaneurysms. Finally, the macula should be examined for the pigmentary changes of age related macular degeneration and the exudates of diabetic maculopathy.

THE RED EYE

The "red eye" is one of the commonest ophthalmic problems presenting to the general practitioner. An accurate history is important and should pay particular attention to vision, the degree and type of discomfort, and the presence of a discharge. The history, together with a good examination, will permit the diagnosis to be made in most cases without recourse to specialist ophthalmic equipment.

Symptoms and signs

The patient's symptoms give many clues to the cause of the red eye. The most important are pain and visual loss, which suggest serious conditions such as corneal ulceration, iritis, and acute glaucoma. A purulent discharge suggests a bacterial conjunctivitis, whereas a clear discharge suggests a viral or allergic cause. A gritty sensation is common in conjunctivitis, but the presence of a foreign body must be excluded, particularly if only one eye is affected. **Corneal abrasions will be missed if fluorescein is not used**.

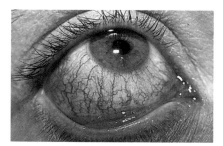

Bacterial conjunctivitis without discharge.

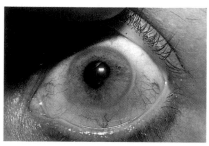

Anterior uveitis with ciliary flush around cornea and irregular stuck down pupil.

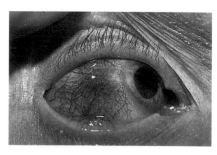

Scleritis.

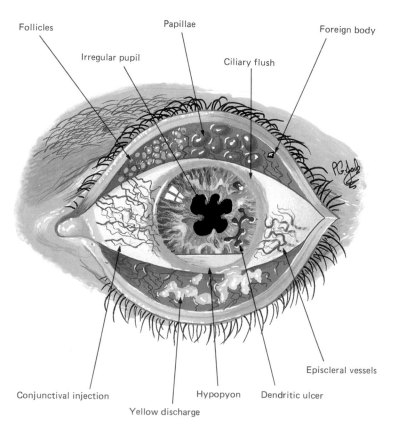

Important physical signs to look for in a patient with a red eye.

Follicles — *Irregular pupil* — *Papillae* — *Ciliary flush* — *Foreign body* — *Conjunctival injection* — *Yellow discharge* — *Hypopyon* — *Dendritic ulcer* — *Episcleral vessels*

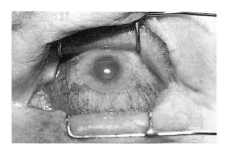

Acute angle closure glaucoma with red eye, semidilated pupil, and hazy cornea.

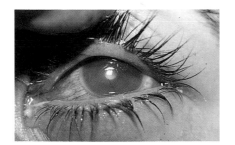

Corneal abscess (pseudomonas) in contact lens wearer.

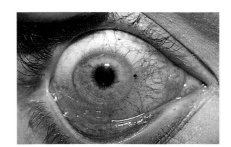

Foreign body.

Conjunctivitis

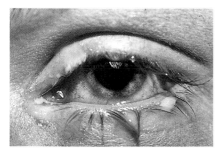

Purulent bacterial conjunctivitis.

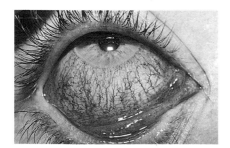

Viral conjunctivitis.

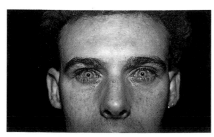

Chlamydial conjunctivitis.

Conjunctivitis is one of the commonest causes of an uncomfortable red eye. Conjunctivitis itself has many causes, including bacteria, viruses, chlamydia, and allergies.

Bacterial conjunctivitis

History—The patient usually has discomfort and a purulent discharge in one eye that characteristically spreads to the other eye. The eye may be difficult to open in the morning because the discharge gums the lashes together. There may be a history of contact with a person with similar symptoms.

Examination—The vision should be normal after the discharge has been blinked clear of the cornea. The discharge is usually mucopurulent and there is uniform engorgement of all the conjunctival blood vessels. There is no staining of the cornea with fluorescein.

Management—Chloramphenicol eye drops should be instilled hourly for 24 hours, decreasing to four times a day, and chloramphenicol ointment applied each night for a week to hasten recovery. Gel preparations of antibiotics which need to be applied less frequently may be more convenient. Patients should be advised about general hygienic measures—for example, not sharing face towels.

Viral conjunctivitis

Viral conjunctivitis is commonly associated with upper respiratory tract infections and is usually caused by an adenovirus. It is the type of conjunctivitis that occurs in epidemics (pink eye).

History—The patient normally complains of both eyes being gritty and uncomfortable. There may be associated symptoms of a cold and cough. The discharge is usually watery. This type of conjunctivitis usually lasts longer than bacterial conjunctivitis and may go on for many weeks. Photophobia and discomfort may be severe if the patient goes on to develop discrete corneal opacities.

Examination—Both eyes are red with diffuse conjunctival injection and there may be a clear discharge. Small white lymphoid aggregations may be present on the conjunctiva (follicles). Small corneal opacities may give rise to pronounced symptoms, but these are difficult to see without high magnification.

Treatment—Viral conjunctivitis is generally a self limiting condition, but chloramphenicol eye drops and ointment provide symptomatic relief and may help prevent secondary bacterial infection. Viral conjunctivitis is extremely contagious and strict hygienic measures are important for both the patient and the doctor—for example, washing of hands, sterilising of instruments, and so on. In view of the chronic course of some cases the patient may return for further treatment, but steroids must not be given without ophthalmological supervision.

Chlamydial conjunctivitis

History—Patients are usually young with a history of chronic bilateral conjunctivitis with a mucopurulent discharge. There may be associated symptoms of venereal disease.

Examination—There is bilateral diffuse conjunctival injection with a

The red eye

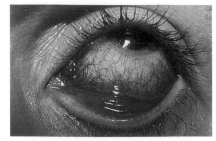

Viral conjunctivitis.

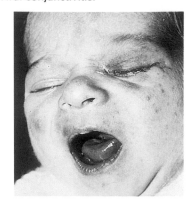

Infantile conjunctivitis

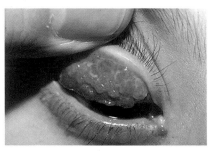

Large papillae in allergic conjunctivitis.

• **Prolonged use of topical steroids can cause glaucoma and cataracts**

---

mucopurulent discharge and many lymphoid aggregates in the conjunctiva (follicles). The cornea is usually inflamed (keratitis) and an infiltrate of the upper cornea (pannus) may be seen.

Management—The diagnosis is often difficult, and special bacteriological tests may be necessary to confirm the clinical suspicions. Treatment comprises tetracycline ointment and oral tetracycline 250 mg four times a day for at least a month. Associated venereal disease should also be treated. World wide, trachoma is one of the major causes of blindness. In developing countries infection by *Chlamydia trachomatis* results in severe scarring of the conjunctiva and the underlying tarsal plate. The eyelids turn in and permanently scar the already damaged cornea.

Conjunctivitis in infants

Conjunctivitis in young children is extremely important because the eye defences are immature and a severe conjunctivitis with membrane formation and bleeding may occur. Serious corneal disease and blindness may result. Conjunctivitis in an infant less than 1 month old (ophthalmia neonatorum) is a notifiable disease. Such babies must be seen in an eye department so that special cultures can be taken and appropriate treatment given. Venereal disease in the parents must be excluded.

Allergic conjunctivitis

History—The main feature is itching. Both eyes are usually affected and there may be a clear discharge. There may be a family history of atopy or recent contact with chemicals or eye drops. Similar symptoms may have occurred at the same time in previous years.

Examination—The conjunctivae are diffusely injected and may be oedematous (chemosis). The discharge is clear and stringy. Because of the fibrous septa that tether the eyelid (tarsal) conjunctivae, oedema results in round swellings (papillae). When these are large they are referred to as cobblestones.

Treatment—Topical antihistamine and vasoconstrictor eye drops provide short term relief. Sodium cromoglycate eye drops prevent degranulation of mast cells but they may need to be used for several weeks to achieve maximal effect and patients should be advised to persist with the drops if relief is not immediate. Oral antihistamines may also be used, particularly the newer compounds that cause less sedation. Topical steroids are effective, but should not be used for long without ophthalmological supervision because of the risk of steroid induced cataracts and glaucoma.

Episcleritis and scleritis

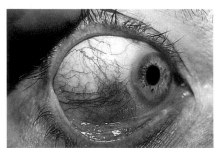

Episcleritis.

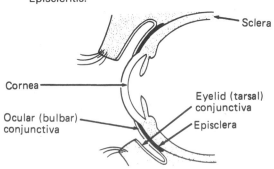

Conjunctiva, sclera, and episclera.

Episcleritis and scleritis differ from conjunctivitis in that they usually present as a *localised* area of inflammation. The episclera lies just beneath the conjunctiva and adjacent to the tough white scleral coat of the eye. Both the sclera and episclera may become inflamed, particularly in rheumatoid arthritis and other autoimmune conditions, but no cause is found for most cases of episcleritis. Episcleritis is essentially self limiting; scleritis is much more serious and complications include ocular perforations.

History–The patient complains of a red and sore eye that may also be tender. There may be reflex lacrimation but usually no discharge. Scleritis is much more painful than episcleritis.

Examination–There is a localised area of inflammation that is tender to the touch. The episcleral and scleral vessels are larger than the conjunctival vessels. Scleritis is characteristically much more painful than episcleritis, and the signs of inflammation are usually more florid.

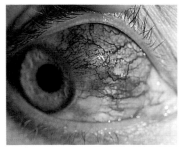

Scleritis.

Management—Any underlying cause should be identified. Although episcleritis is essentially self limiting, steroid eye drops hasten recovery and provide symptomatic relief. Scleritis is much more serious, and all patients need ophthalmological review. Serious systemic disorders should be excluded, and systemic immunosuppressive treatment may be required.

Corneal ulceration

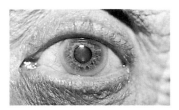

Eye with herpes simplex ulcer (not visible without fluorescein).

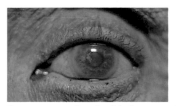

Same eye stained with fluorescein and viewed with blue light (ulcer visible).

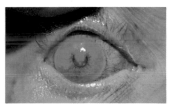

Herpes simplex ulcers inadvertently treated with steroids. Ulceration has spread and grown.

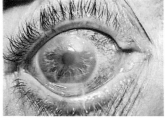

Corneal abscess with pus in anterior chamber (hypopyon).

Corneal ulcers may be caused by bacterial, viral, and fungal infections; these may occur as primary events or be secondary to an event that has compromised the eye—for example, abrasion, contact lens wear, or use of topical steroids.

History—Pain is a prominent feature as the cornea is an exquisitely sensitive organ, though this is not so when corneal sensation is impaired—for example, after herpes zoster ophthalmicus. Indeed, this lack of sensation may be the cause of the ulceration. There may be clues such as similar past attacks, facial cold sores, a recent abrasion, or the wearing of contact lenses.

Examination—Visual acuity depends on the location and size of the ulcer, and normal visual acuity does not exclude an ulcer. There may be a watery discharge due to reflex lacrimation, or a mucopurulent discharge in bacterial ulcers. Conjunctival injection may be generalised or localised if the ulcer is peripheral, giving a clue to its presence. Fluorescein must be used or an ulcer may easily be missed. Certain types of corneal ulceration are characteristic. If there is inflammation in the anterior chamber there may be a collection of pus present (hypopyon). The upper eyelid must be everted or a subtarsal foreign body causing corneal ulceration may be missed. Patients with subtarsal foreign bodies sometimes do not recollect anything entering the eye.

Management—Patients with corneal ulceration should be referred urgently to an eye department or the sight may be lost. Management depends on the cause of the ulceration. The diagnosis may usually be made on the clinical appearance. The appropriate swabs and cultures should be arranged to try to identify the causative organism. Intensive treatment is then started with drops and ointment of broad spectrum antibiotics until the organisms and their sensitivities are known. Injection of antibiotics into the subconjunctival space may be given to increase local concentrations of the drugs. Cycloplegic drops are used to relieve pain due to spasm of the ciliary muscle, and as they are also mydriatics (dilate the pupil) they prevent adhesions of the iris to the lens (posterior synechiae). Systemic steroids may be used to reduce local inflammatory damage not caused by direct infection, but the indications for their use are specific and they should not be used without ophthalmological supervision.

Iritis, iridocyclitis, and anterior uveitis

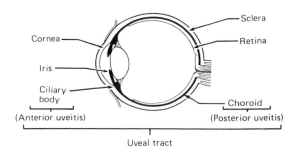

The iris, ciliary body, and choroid are embryologically similar and are known as the uveal tract. Inflammation of the iris (iritis) does not occur without inflammation of the ciliary body (cyclitis) and together these are referred to as iridocyclitis, or anterior uveitis. Thus the terms are synonymous.

Several groups of patients are at risk, including those who have had past attacks of iritis, and those with a seronegative arthropathy, particularly if they are positive for the HLA-B27 histocompatability antigen—for example, a young man with ankylosing spondylitis.

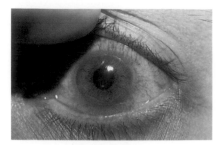

Anterior uveitis/iritis with ciliary flush but pupil not stuck down.

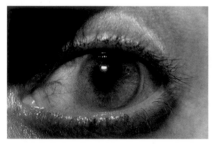

Anterior uveitis with ciliary flush and irregular pupil.

Acute angle closure glaucoma

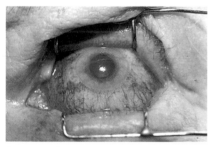

Acute angle closure glaucoma. Note the corneal oedema (irregular reflected image of light on cornea) and fixed semi-dilated pupil.

Features

- Pain
- Haloes round lights
- Impaired vision
- Fixed semidilated pupil
- Hazy cornea
- Age > 50
- Eye feels hard
- Unilateral

Children with seronegative arthritis are also at high risk, particularly if they have only a few joints affected by the arthritis. Their uveitis may be relatively asymptomatic and they may suffer serious ocular damage if they are not screened. Other causes of chronic anterior uveitis include sarcoidosis and several infections including herpes zoster ophthalmicus, syphilis, and tuberculosis.

History—The patient who has had past attacks can often feel an attack coming on before physical signs are present. There is often pain in the later stages, with photophobia due to inflammation and ciliary spasm. The pain may be worse when the patient is reading and contracting the ciliary muscle.

Examination—The vision may initially be normal but later it may be impaired. Accommodation may be affected, there may be inflammatory cells in the anterior chamber, cataracts may form, and adhesions may develop between the iris and the lens. The affected eye is red with the injection being particularly pronounced over the area covering the inflamed ciliary body (ciliary flush). The pupil is small because of spasm of the sphincter or irregular because of adhesions of the iris to the lens (posterior synechiae). An abnormal pupil in a red eye usually indicates serious ocular disease. Inflammatory cells may be deposited on the back of the cornea (keratitic precipitates) or may settle to form a collection of cells in the anterior chamber of the eye (hypopyon).

Management—If there is an underlying cause it must be treated, but in many cases no cause is found. It is important to ensure that there is no disease in the rest of the eye that is giving rise to signs of an anterior uveitis such as more posterior inflammation, a retinal detachment, or an intraocular tumour. Treatment is with topical steroids to reduce the inflammation and prevent adhesions within the eye. The ciliary body is paralysed to relieve pain, and the associated dilatation of the pupil also helps to prevent the development of adhesions between the iris and lens that can cause "pupil block" glaucoma. The intraocular pressure may also rise because inflammatory cells block the trabecular meshwork, and pressure lowering treatment may have to be given if this occurs. Continued inflammation may lead to permanent damage of the trabecular meshwork, cataracts, and oedema of the macula.

Acute glaucoma should always be considered in a patient over the age of 50 with a painful red eye. The diagnosis must not be missed or the eye will be permanently damaged. The mechanism is dealt with in the chapter on the glaucomas.

History—The attack usually comes on quite quickly, characteristically in the evening when the pupil becomes semidilated. There is pain in one eye, which can be extremely severe and may be accompanied by vomiting. The patient complains of impaired vision and haloes around lights due to oedema of the cornea. The patient may have had similar attacks in the past that were relieved by going to sleep (the pupil constricts during sleep, so relieving the attack).

Examination—The eye is inflamed and tender. The cornea is hazy and the pupil is semidilated and fixed. Vision is impaired according to the state of the cornea. On gentle palpation the eye feels harder than the other eye. The anterior chamber seems shallower than usual, with the iris being close to the cornea. If the patient is seen after the resolution of an attack the signs may have disappeared—hence the importance of the history.

Management—Urgent referral to hospital is required. Emergency treatment is needed if the sight in the eye is to be preserved. If it is not possible to get the patient to an eye hospital straight away, intravenous acetazolamide (Diamox) 500 mg should be given, and pilocarpine 4% should be instilled in the eye to constrict the pupil. The pressure must first be brought down medically and a hole then made in the iris surgically (iridectomy) or with a laser (iridotomy) to restore normal aqueous flow. The other eye should be treated prophylactically in a similar way. If treatment is delayed adhesions may form between the iris and the cornea (peripheral anterior synechiae) or the trabecular meshwork may be permanently damaged, necessitating a full surgical drainage procedure.

EYELID AND LACRIMAL DISORDERS

Lumps in the lid

Importance

- May need disfiguring operations if left
- May be life threatening
- May be the cause of visual disturbance
- May cause blindness in children
- May indicate systemic disease

The commonest lump found in the eyelid is a chalazion, but the accurate diagnosis of a lid lump is important because the lump:
- May necessitate a disfiguring operation if not treated early—basal cell carcinoma
- May be life threatening—a deep invading basal cell carcinoma
- May be the cause of visual disturbance—a chalazion pressing on the cornea and causing astigmatism
- May indicate systemic disease—xanthelasmas in a patient with hyperlipidaemia
- May cause amblyopia if it obstructs vision in a young child.

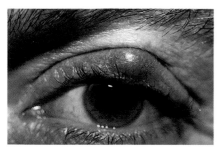

Chalazion.

Chalazion

A chalazion (meibomian cyst) is a granuloma of the lipid secreting meibomian glands that lie in the lid. It is probably the result of a blocked duct with local reaction to the accumulation of lipid. The patient may initially complain of a lump in the lid that is hard and inflamed. This settles and the patient is left with a discrete lump in the lid that may give rise to astigmatism and consequent blurring of vision. Clinically there is a hard lump in the lid, which is clearly visible when the lid is everted.

Many chalazia settle on conservative treatment. This comprises hot compresses (with a towel soaked in warm water) and the application of chloramphenicol ointment. If the chalazion is uncomfortable, excessively large, persistent, or disturbing vision it can be incised and curetted under local anaesthesia from the inner conjunctival side of the eyelid. Recurrent chalazia may suggest an underlying problem such as blepharitis, a skin disorder such as acne rosacea, or very rarely a malignant tumour of the meibomian glands.

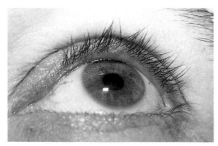

Stye.

Stye

A stye and chalazion are often confused. A stye is an infection of a lash follicle. The patient complains of a red, tender swelling at the lid margin. Unlike a chalazion, there may be a "head" of pus. It should be treated with hot compresses to help it to discharge, and chloramphenicol ointment should be used.

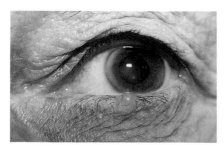

Cyst of sweat secreting gland (cyst of Moll).

Marginal cysts

Marginal cysts may develop from the lipid and sweat secreting glands round the margins of the eyelids. They are dome shaped with no inflammation. The cysts of the sweat glands are filled with clear fluid (cyst of Moll) and the cysts of the lipid secreting glands are filled with yellowish contents (cyst of Zeiss).

If they are not causing any problems no treatment is indicated. If they are a cosmetic blemish they can be removed under local anaesthetic.

Eyelid and lacrimal disorders

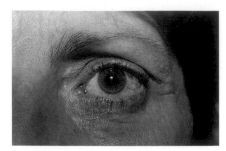

Xanthelasmas and corneal arcus in a young patient.

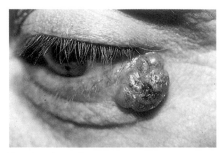

Basal cell carcinoma.

Papilloma

Papillomas are often pedunculated and multilobular. They are common and may be caused by viruses. They should be removed if they are large and the diagnosis is uncertain, or if they are disfiguring.

Xanthelasma

Xanthelasmas may be an incidental finding, or the patient may complain of yellow plaques on the nasal side of the eyelids; these contain lipid. Associated hyperlipidaemia must be excluded and the lesions may be removed under local anaesthetic if they cause a cosmetic problem.

Basal cell carcinoma

Basal cell carcinoma (rodent ulcer) is the most common malignant tumour of the eyelid, and it occurs mainly in the lower lid, which is particularly exposed to sunlight. Though it does not metastasise, it may be life threatening if allowed to infiltrate locally. If it is large by the time the patient is referred an extensive and often disfiguring operation may be necessary.

The classic basal cell carcinoma has a pearly rounded edge with a necrotic centre, but it may be difficult to diagnose if it presents as a diffuse indurated lesion. It is particularly easy to miss the invasive form that occurs in a skin crease, which may be invading deeply with few cutaneous signs.

The patient should be referred urgently if there is any suspicion of a basal cell carcinoma. It is usually excised under local anaesthesia, unless complicated plastic surgery is required. Radiotherapy may also be used.

Inflammatory diseases of the eyelid

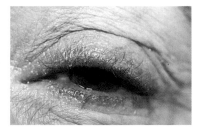

Blepharitis.

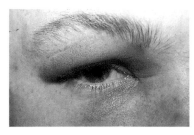

Inflammation of upper eyelid after expression of blackhead.

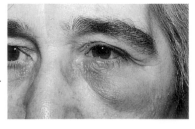

Chalazion with associated inflammation of lower eyelid.

Blepharitis

Blepharitis is a common condition but is often not diagnosed. It is a chronic disease; the patient complains of persistently sore eyes. The symptoms may be intermittent and include a gritty sensation and sore eyelids. The patient may present with a chalazion or stye, which are much more common in patients with blepharitis, and these may be recurrent. Physical signs include inflamed lid margins, blocked meibomian gland orifices, and crusts round the lid margins. The conjunctiva may be inflamed, and punctate staining of the cornea may be visible on staining with fluorescein. Associated skin diseases include rosacea, eczema, and psoriasis. The aims of treatment are to:

- *Keep the lids clean*—the crusts and coagulated lipid should be gently cleaned with a cotton wool bud dipped in warm water
- *Treat infection*—antibiotic ointment should be smeared on the lid margin to help kill the staphylococci in the eyelid that may be aggravating the condition; this may be done for several months
- *Replace tears*—the tear film in patients with blepharitis is abnormal, and artificial tears may provide considerable relief of symptoms
- *Treat sebaceous gland dysfunction*—in severe cases or those associated with sebaceous gland dysfunction, such as rosacea, oral tetracycline may be invaluable. Indications for referral are poor response to treatment and corneal disease.

Acute inflammation of the eyelid

It is important to achieve a diagnosis in a patient with an acutely inflamed eyelid as some conditions may be blinding—for example, orbital cellulitis. There are several causes.

- *A chalazion or stye*—Routine treatment should be given for these conditions. In addition, if infection is spreading systemic antibiotics may be indicated.

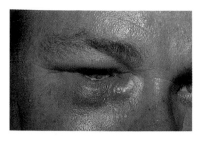

Dacryocystitis.

Orbital cellulitis can cause blindness if not treated immediately—particularly in children

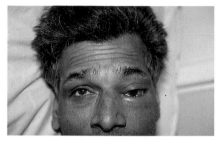

Orbital cellulitis: swollen eyelids, conjunctival swelling, displaced eyeball, and restricted eye movements.

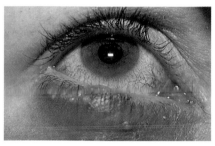

Herpes simplex with associated conjunctivitis.

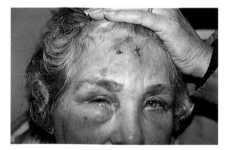

Herpes zoster ophthalmicus with swollen eyelids.

● *Spread of local infection*—This may be from a local lesion such as a "squeezed" comedo. Again if there is spread of infection systemic antibiotics are indicated.

● *Acute dacryocystitis*—The site of inflammation is medial, over the lacrimal sac. There may be a history of previous watering of the eye due to a blocked lacrimal system that has since become infected. Treatment is with topical chloramphenicol and systemic antibiotics until the infection resolves. Recurrent attacks or symptomatic watering of the eye are indications for operation.

● *Orbital cellulitis*—This is a potentially blinding and life threatening condition that must not be missed. It usually results from the spread of infection from adjacent sinuses. It is particularly important in children, in whom blindness may ensue in hours. The patient usually presents with unilateral swollen eyelids that may not be red. Features to look for include:

> **The patient is unwell**
> **There is tenderness over the sinuses**
> **There is restriction of eye movements.**

The possibility of orbital cellulitis should always be kept in mind, especially in children, and patients should be referred immediately.

● *Allergy*—There may be a history of contact with an allergen, including animals, plants, chemicals, or cosmetics. Itching is a good indicator of allergy, and the allergen should be avoided. Treatment may include the application of a weak topical steroid ointment—for example, hydrocortisone 1%—for a short period.

● *Herpes simplex* may present as a vesicular rash on the skin of the eyelid. There may be associated areas of vesicular eruption on the face. An "experienced" patient may be able to discern the prodromal tingling sensation. Early application of acyclovir cream will shorten the length and severity of the episode. Associated ocular herpetic disease should be considered if the eye is red, and the patient should then be referred immediately.

● *Herpes zoster ophthalmicus* (shingles) presents as a vesicular rash over the distribution of the ophthalmic division of the fifth cranial nerve. There may be associated pain and the patient usually feels unwell. The eye is often affected, particularly if the side of the nose is also affected (which is innervated by a branch of the nasociliary nerve that also innervates the eye). Common ocular problems include conjunctivitis, keratitis, and uveitis. The eye is often shut because of oedema of the eyelid, but an attempt should be made to inspect the globe. If the eye is red or if there is visual disturbance the patient should be referred straight away. The ocular complications of herpes zoster may occur late in the disease so the eye should be examined at each visit. Treatment includes application of a wetting cream after crusting, to prevent painful and disfiguring scars. If the eye is affected topical antibiotics may prevent secondary infection, and acyclovir ointment is used. Oral acyclovir given early in the course of the disease may reduce the incidence of long term sequelae, such as pain.

Malpositions of the eyelids and eyelashes

Main symptoms:

● Irritation of the eye by lashes rubbing on it (entropion)
● Watering of the eye caused by malposition of the punctum (ectropion)

Malpositions of the eyelids and eyelashes are common and give rise to various symptoms, including irritation of the eye by lashes rubbing on it (entropion and ingrowing eyelashes) and watering of the eye caused by malposition of the punctum (ectropion). The eyelids are folds of skin with fibrous plates in both the upper and lower lids, and the circular muscle (orbicularis) controls the closing of the eyes. Any change in the muscles or supporting tissues may result in malposition of the lids.

Eyelid and lacrimal disorders

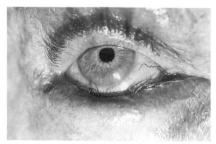

Entropion. Inturning eyelashes may scratch and damage the cornea.

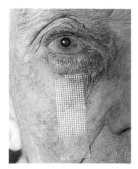

Temporary treatment of entropion.

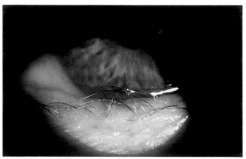

Trichiasis.

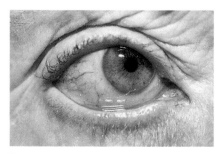

Ectropion with resulting epiphora.

Ptosis may occasionally:

- Indicate a life threatening disease
- Indicate a systemic disease
- Cause amblyopia in children

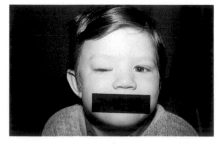

Ptosis caused by lid haemangioma: exclude amblyopia in a child.

Entropion

The patient may present complaining of irritation due to the eyelashes rubbing on the cornea. This may be immediately apparent on examination but may be intermittent, in which case the lid may be in the normal position. The clue is that the eyelashes of the lower lid are pushed to the side by the regular inturning, and the cornea should be examined by staining with fluorescein. The entropion can be brought on by asking the patient to close the eyes tightly, and then open the eyes. Entropion is common, particularly in elderly patients with some spasm of the eyelids. The great danger of entropion is ulceration and scarring of the cornea by the abrading eyelashes. Temporary treatment consists of taping down the lower lid and applying chloramphenicol ointment. An operation under local anaesthesia is required to correct the entropion permanently. Scarring of the cornea associated with entropion due to trachoma is one of the commonest causes of blindness on a worldwide scale.

Trichiasis

Sometimes the lid may be in a normal position, but aberrant eyelashes may grow inwards. This is more common in the presence of diseases of the eyelid such as blepharitis or trachoma. The lashes can be seen on examination, especially with magnification. They can be pulled out, but they frequently regrow. The application of chloramphenicol ointment helps to prevent corneal damage, and electrolysis of the hair roots or cryotherapy may be necessary to stop the lashes regrowing.

Ectropion

The initial complaint may be that of a watery eye. The tears drain mainly through the lower punctum at the medial end of the lower lid. If the eyelid is not properly apposed to the eye tears cannot flow into the punctum, and the result is a watery eye. The patient may also complain of the unsightly appearance of an ectropion. The most common reason for ectropion is laxity of the tissues of the lid due to aging, but it also occurs if the muscles are lax as in the case of a facial nerve palsy. Scarring of the skin of the eyelid may also pull the lid margin down. Ectropion can be rectified by an operation under local anaesthesia. Before operation the use of ointment will help to protect the eye and prevent drying of the exposed conjunctiva.

Ptosis

Ptosis or drooping of the eyelid may:

- Indicate a life threatening condition such as a third nerve palsy secondary to an aneurysm, or a Horner's syndrome secondary to carcinoma of the lung.

- Indicate a disease that needs systemic treatment such as myasthenia gravis.

- Cause irreversible amblyopia in a child due to the lid obstructing vision. If there is any question of a ptosis obstructing vision in a child he or she should be urgently referred.

- Be easily treatable by a simple operation (senile ptosis).

The patient will usually complain of a drooping eyelid. The upper eyelid is raised by the levator muscle, which is controlled by the third nerve. There is also Müller's muscle, which is controlled by the sympathetic nervous system. These are attached to the fibrous plate in the eyelid and other lid structures. The ptosis can occur because of defects in:

Lid tissues—With aging the tissues become lax and the connections loosen, resulting in ptosis; this is common in the elderly. The eye movements and pupils should be normal. A pseudoptosis may occur when the eyelid skin sags and droops down over the lid margin. Both these conditions are amenable to relatively simple operations under local anaesthesia.

Muscle tissue—It is important not to miss a general muscular disorder such as myasthenia gravis or dystrophia myotonica. Any diplopia, worsening symptoms throughout the day, and other muscular symptoms should lead one to suspect myasthenia. The patient's facies and handshake may give clues to the diagnosis of dystrophia myotonica.

Nerve supply—A third nerve palsy may present as a ptosis. This, together with an abducted eye and dilated pupil, indicates the diagnosis. The patient should be urgently referred as causes include a compressive lesion of the third nerve such as an aneurysm. Diabetes should be excluded.

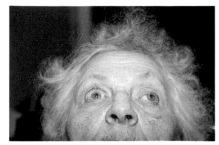

Left ptosis caused by pupil sparing third nerve palsy.

Horner's syndrome due to damage to the sympathetic chain—The pupil is small but reactive, and sweating over that side of the face may be reduced. The eye movements should be normal. Causes include lesions of the brain stem and spinal cord, and apical lung tumours, so the patient should be referred.

The lacrimal system

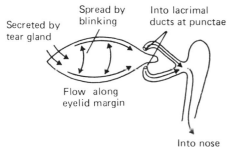

Normal tear flow.

Secreted by tear gland · Spread by blinking · Into lacrimal ducts at punctae · Flow along eyelid margin · Into nose

The watering eye

Tears are produced by the lacrimal gland that lies in the upper lateral aspect of the orbit. They flow down across the eye along the lid margins and are spread across the eye by blinking. They then flow through the upper and lower puncta to the lacrimal sac and down the nasolacrimal duct into the nose. A watering eye may occur for several reasons.

- *Excessive production of tears*—This is rare, but can occur paradoxically in a patient with "dry eyes". Basal secretion of tears is inadequate and this results in drying of the eye. This gives rise to a reactive secretion of tears, which causes epiphora. The patient may give a history of intermittent discomfort followed by watering of the eye.

- *Punctal malposition secondary to lid malposition*—The puncta must be well apposed to the eye to drain tears. Even mild ectropion can result in pooling of tears and overflow. Careful examination of the lid will usually show any malposition, which can be remedied by performing a minor operation.

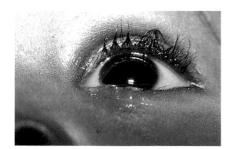

Blocked left nasolacrimal system in a child.

- *Punctal stenosis*—The puncta may close up and this will result in watering. If this is the case the puncta cannot be seen easily on examination with a magnifying loupe. They can be surgically dilated or opened by a minor operation under local anaesthesia.

- *Blockage of the lacrimal sac or nasolacrimal duct*—If the nasolacrimal duct is blocked and cannot be freed by syringing an operation may be required to bypass the obstruction. A common operation for this is dacryocystorhinostomy, in which a hole is made through into the nose from the sac and sometimes plastic tubes are left in for several months to create a fistula. This is a major operation and usually performed under general anaesthesia.

In children the lacrimal drainage system may not be patent. The child may present with a watering eye or sometimes with recurrent conjunctivitis. Treatment is usually with chloramphenicol eye drops, and the mother should be advised to massage the lacrimal sac to encourage flow. If the watering persists, the child may have to have the

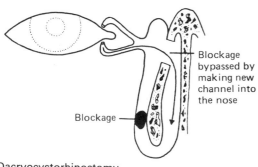

Blockage · Blockage bypassed by making new channel into the nose

Dacryocystorhinostomy.

Eyelid and lacrimal disorders

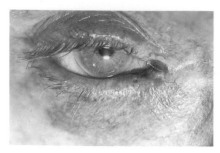

Watering eye caused by punctal ectropion.

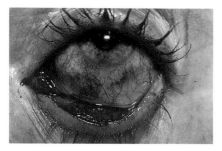

Dry eye in rheumatoid arthritis stained with rose bengal drops.

sac and duct probed under general anaesthesia. If the blockage persists a dacryocystorhinostomy may be performed when the child is older, but this is not often necessary.

The dry eye

The dry eye is common in the elderly, in whom tear secretion is reduced. The patient usually presents complaining of a chronic gritty sensation in the eye, which is not particularly red. Systemic diseases such as rheumatoid arthritis are associated with a dry eye. Drugs such as diuretics may also exacerbate the symptoms of a dry eye. Staining of the cornea may be apparent with fluorescein and rose bengal drops. If rose bengal eye drops are used the eyes must be washed out very thoroughly as these drops are a potent irritant. Treatment includes:

- *Artificial tear drops*, which may be used as frequently as necessary
- *Simple ointment*, which helps to give prolonged lubrication, particularly at night when tear secretion is minimal
- *Acetylcysteine eye drops*, which are useful if there is clumping of mucus on the eye (filamentary keratitis), but many patients find that the drops sting
- *Treatment* of any associated blepharitis.

INJURIES TO THE EYE

History

- Corneal abrasions
- Foreign bodies
- Radiation damage
- Chemical damage
- Blunt injuries
- Penetrating injuries

An injury to the eye or its surrounding tissues is the commonest reason for attendance at the eye casualty department.

The history of how the injury was sustained is crucial as it gives clues to what should be looked for during the examination. **If there is a story of any high velocity injury (particularly a hammer and chisel injury) a penetrating injury must be strongly suspected, and excluded.** If there has been a forceful blunt injury (such as a punch) signs of a "blow out" fracture should be sought. The circumstances of the injury must be elicited and carefully recorded as these may have important medicolegal implications.

Examination

A good examination is vital if there is a history of eye injury. Specific signs must be sought or they will be missed. These are illustrated below. It is vital to test visual acuity both to establish a baseline value and to alert the examiner to the possibility of further problems, although an acuity of 6/6 does not necessarily exclude serious problems—even a penetrating injury. The visual acuity may also have considerable medicolegal implications. Local anaesthetic may need to be used to obtain a good view, and the use of fluorescein is mandatory if an abrasion is not to be missed.

The injured eye

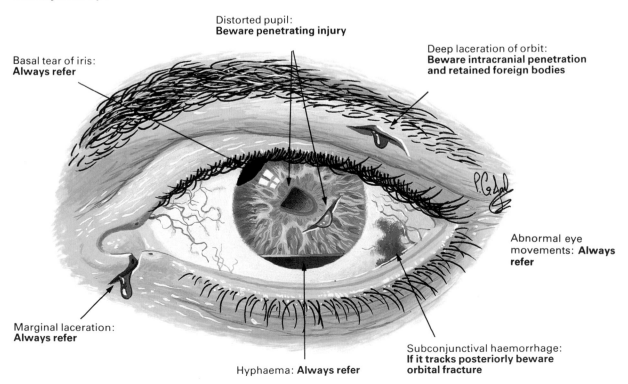

Distorted pupil:
Beware penetrating injury

Deep laceration of orbit:
Beware intracranial penetration and retained foreign bodies

Basal tear of iris:
Always refer

Abnormal eye movements: **Always refer**

Marginal laceration:
Always refer

Hyphaema: **Always refer**

Subconjunctival haemorrhage:
If it tracks posteriorly beware orbital fracture

Corneal abrasions

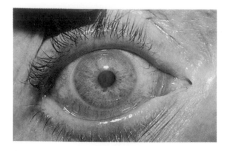

Corneal abrasion stained with fluorescein and illuminated with white light.

Corneal abrasions are the commonest consequence of blunt injury. They may follow injuries with foreign bodies, fingernails, or twigs. **Abrasions will be missed if fluorescein is not instilled.** The aims of treatment are:
- *To speed healing and protect the eye*—pad the eye.
- *To prevent infection*—apply chloramphenicol ointment.
- *To relieve pain*—instil a cycloplegic (homatropine 2%); give oral analgesia if necessary.

The drops will relieve ciliary spasm and also dilate the pupil. The patient uses an eye pad for a day or so until the abrasion heals. An eye pad may not be necessary for small abrasions. Chloramphenicol drops can be used for a few more days to help prevent any infection and lubricate the eye.

Recurrent abrasions—Occasionally the epithelium of the cornea may repeatedly break down in an area where there has been a previous injury or where there is an inherently weak adhesion between the epithelial cells and the basement membrane. The recurrences usually occur at night when there is little secretion of tears and the epithelium may be torn off. Treatment is long term and entails using tear drops during the day and ointment at night to lubricate the eye. An operation to enhance the adhesion between the epithelium and the underlying basement membrane may occasionally be necessary.

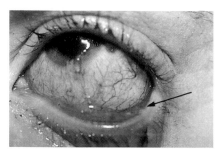

Corneal abrasion stained with fluorescein and illuminated with blue light.

Foreign bodies

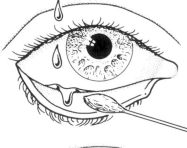

Lower lid gently pulled down to show a conjunctival foreign body. The cornea has also been perforated.

It is important to identify and remove conjunctival and corneal foreign bodies as soon as possible. A patient may not recall a foreign body having entered the eye, so it is essential to exclude a foreign body if a patient has an uncomfortable red eye. It may be necessary to use local anaesthetic both to examine the eye and to remove the foreign body. Although patients often request them, local anaesthetics should never be given to the patient to use because they impede healing, and further injury may occur to an anaesthetised eye.

Small loose conjunctival foreign bodies can be removed with the edge of a tissue or a cotton wool bud, or they can be washed out with water. The upper lid must be everted to exclude a subtarsal foreign body, particularly if there are corneal scratches or the continuing feeling that a foreign body is present. Corneal foreign bodies are often more difficult to remove and if they are metallic are often "rusted on." They must be removed as they will prevent healing and the rust may permanently stain the cornea. A cotton wool bud or the edge of a piece of cardboard may be used. If this does not work a needle tip (or a special rotary drill) can be used, but great care must be taken when using these as the eye may easily be damaged. If there is any doubt, these patients should be referred to an ophthalmic surgeon. When the foreign body has been removed any remaining epithelial defect can be treated as an abrasion.

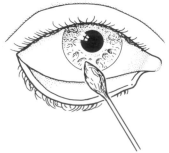

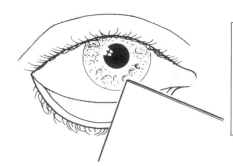

Removal of a foreign body

- **Use local anaesthetic**
- If it is loose, irrigate
- If it is adherent, use a cotton wool bud or a piece of cardboard.

Radiation damage

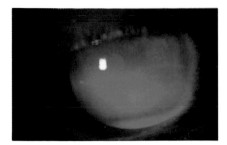

Cornea after welding damage stained with fluorescein and illuminated with blue light.

The commonest form of radiation damage occurs when welding has been carried out without adequate shielding of the eye. The corneal epithelium is damaged by the ultraviolet rays and the patient typically presents with painful, weeping eyes some hours after welding. Radiation damage can also occur after exposure to large amounts of reflected sunlight—for example, snow blindness. Treatment is as for a corneal abrasion.

Chemical damage

- Wash out immediately
- Remove loose particles
- Refer to ophthalmic department
- **BEWARE ALKALIS**

If chemicals are splashed into the eye the eye and the conjunctival sacs (fornices) should immediately be washed out with copious amounts of water. Alkalis are particularly damaging, and any loose bits such as lime should be removed from the fornices with the aid of local anaesthetic if necessary. The patient should then be referred immediately to an ophthalmic department. If there is any doubt irrigation should be continued for as long as possible.

Blunt injuries

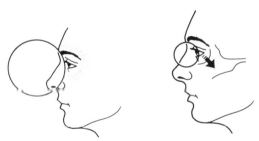

Large object—impact on orbital margin.

Small object—eye and orbit take impact.

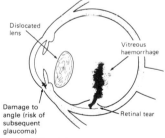

Dislocated lens

Vitreous haemorrhage

Damage to angle (risk of subsequent glaucoma)

Retinal tear

Complications of blunt trauma to the eye.

If a large object (such as a football) hits the eye most of the impact is usually taken by the orbital margin. If a smaller object (such as a squash ball) hits the area the eye itself may take most of the impact. Haemorrhage may occur and a collection of blood may be plainly visible in the anterior chamber of the eye (hyphaema). These patients need to be reviewed at an eye hospital as the pressure in the eye may rise, and further haemorrhages may need to be removed surgically. Haemorrhage may also occur into the vitreous or in the retina, and this may be accompanied by a retinal detachment. All patients with visual impairment after blunt injury should be seen in an ophthalmic department.

The pupil may also be damaged and react poorly to light. This is particularly important in a patient with an associated head injury, as this may be interpreted as—or mask—the dilated pupil that is suggestive of an acute extradural haematoma. The lens may be damaged or dislocated, and a cataract may develop. Damage to the drainage angle of the eye (which cannot be seen without a mirror contact lens and a slit lamp microscope) increases the chances of glaucoma developing in later life. If the force of impact is transmitted to the orbit an orbital fracture may occur (usually in the floor, which is thin and has little support). Clues to the presence of an inferior "blow out" fracture include diplopia, a recessed eye, defective eye movements (especially vertical), an ipsilateral nose bleed, and diminished sensation over the distribution of the infraorbital nerve. The fracture may need repair and these patients should be referred to an ophthalmic department.

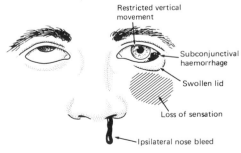

Restricted vertical movement

Subconjunctival haemorrhage

Swollen lid

Loss of sensation

Ipsilateral nose bleed

Signs of a left orbital blowout fracture (patient looking upwards).

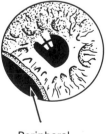

Hyphaema

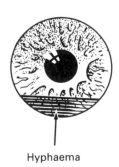

Peripheral tear in iris

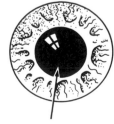

Enlarged pupil: damaged sphincter

Penetrating injuries

Beware:

- Hammer and chisel
- Glass
- Knives
- Thorns
- Darts
- Pencils

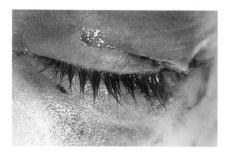

Lacerated eyelid.

Lacerations to the eyelids need specialist attention if:

- *The lid margins have been torn*—these must be sewn together accurately.
- *The lacrimal ducts have been damaged*—the cut ends must be reapposed.
- *There is any suspicion of a foreign body or penetrating eyelid injury*—objects may easily penetrate the orbit and even the cranial cavity through the orbit.

Penetrating injuries of the eye can easily be missed because they may seal themselves, and the signs of abnormality are subtle. Any history of high velocity injury (particularly a hammer and chisel injury) should lead one strongly to suspect a penetrating injury. If there is any suspicion of a penetrating injury the eye should be examined very gently and no pressure should be brought to bear on the globe.

Signs to look for include a distorted pupil, cataract, and vitreous haemorrhage. The pupil should be dilated (if there is no head injury) and a thorough search made for an intraocular foreign body. If in any doubt, a radiograph of the orbit should be taken.

If the eye is clearly perforated it should be protected from any pressure and the patient sent immediately to the nearest eye department.

ACUTE VISUAL DISTURBANCE

Symptoms and signs

Causes and features of acute visual disturbance (in an uninflamed eye)

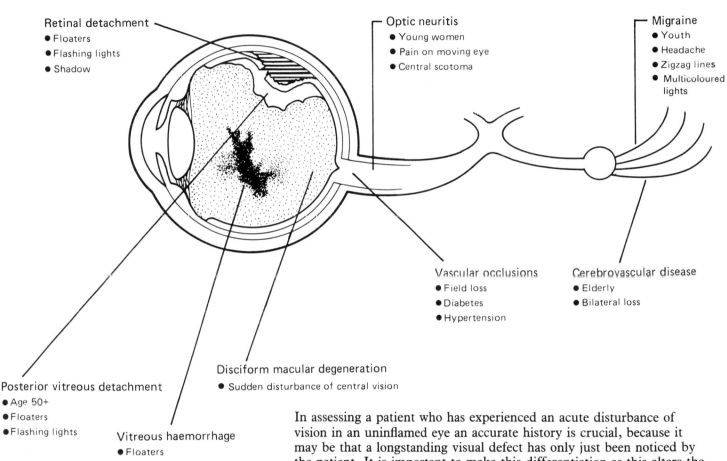

Retinal detachment
- Floaters
- Flashing lights
- Shadow

Optic neuritis
- Young women
- Pain on moving eye
- Central scotoma

Migraine
- Youth
- Headache
- Zigzag lines
- Multicoloured lights

Vascular occlusions
- Field loss
- Diabetes
- Hypertension

Cerebrovascular disease
- Elderly
- Bilateral loss

Disciform macular degeneration
- Sudden disturbance of central vision

Posterior vitreous detachment
- Age 50+
- Floaters
- Flashing lights

Vitreous haemorrhage
- Floaters

History

- Floaters
- Field loss
- Zigzag lines
- Flashing lights
- Headache
- Pain on moving eye

Examination

- Acuity
- Pupil reactions
- Red reflex
- Field loss
- Appearance of retina, macula, and optic nerve

In assessing a patient who has experienced an acute disturbance of vision in an uninflamed eye an accurate history is crucial, because it may be that a longstanding visual defect has only just been noticed by the patient. It is important to make this differentiation as this alters the range of diagnoses and the urgency of treatment. Acute visual disturbance of unknown cause requires urgent referral.

In many cases the diagnosis may be made from the history. Symptoms of floaters or flashing lights suggest a vitreous detachment, a vitreous haemorrhage, or a retinal detachment. Horizontal field loss usually indicates a retinal vascular problem, whereas a vertical defect suggests an abnormality posterior to the optic chiasm. If there is central field loss ("I can't see things in the centre") there may be a disorder at the macula. Associated symptoms such as headache may indicate giant cell arteritis or migraine.

The visual acuity gives a strong clue to the diagnosis. A total lack of perception of light indicates complete occlusion of either the central retinal artery or the arteries supplying the head of the optic nerve. The nature of the field defect gives clues as outlined above. Obstruction of the red reflex on ophthalmoscopy suggests a vitreous haemorrhage, although the patient may have a pre-existing cataract. The appearances of the macula, remaining retina, and head of the optic nerve will indicate the diagnosis if there has been a haemorrhage or arterial or venous occlusion in these areas.

Posterior vitreous detachment

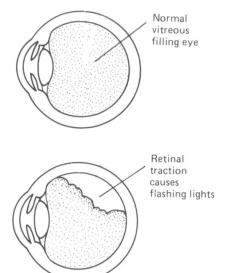

Normal vitreous filling eye

Retinal traction causes flashing lights

Posterior vitreous detachment is the commonest cause of the acute onset of floaters, particularly with advancing age, and is one of the commonest causes of acute visual disturbance.

History—The patient presents complaining of floaters. In posterior vitreous detachment the vitreous body collapses and detaches from the retina. If there are associated flashing lights it suggests that there may be traction on the retina, which may result in a retinal hole and a subsequent retinal detachment.

Examination—The visual acuity is characteristically normal, and there should be no loss of visual field.

Management—If there is any doubt about the precise diagnosis the patient should be referred to an ophthalmologist on the same day so that an associated retinal hole or detachment may be excluded.

Vitreous haemorrhage

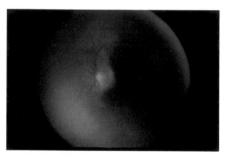

Vitreous haemorrhage.

History—The patient complains of a sudden onset of floaters, or "blobs," in the vision. The visual acuity may be normal or, if the haemorrhage is dense, it may be reduced. Flashing lights indicate retinal traction, which may lead to a retinal hole or detachment. Haemorrhage may occur from spontaneous rupture of vessels, avulsion of vessels during retinal traction, or bleeding from abnormal new vessels. If the patient is shortsighted, retinal detachment is more likely. If there is associated diabetes mellitus the patient may have bled from new vessels.

Examination—The visual acuity depends on the extent of the haemorrhage. Projection of light is accurate unless the haemorrhage is extremely severe. Ophthalmoscopy shows the red reflex to be reduced; there may be clots of blood that move with the vitreous.

Management—The patient should be referred to an ophthalmologist to exclude a retinal detachment. Underlying causes such as diabetes must also be excluded. If a vitreous haemorrhage fails to clear spontaneously the patient may benefit from having the vitreous surgically removed (vitrectomy).

Retinal detachment

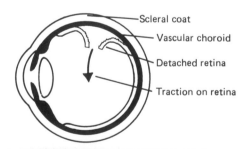

Scleral coat

Vascular choroid

Detached retina

Traction on retina

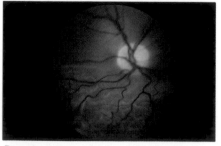

Detached retinal folds—inferior retinal detachment.

Retinal detachment should be suspected from the history. It is only when the detachment is advanced that the vision and the visual fields are affected and the detachment becomes readily visible on direct ophthalmoscopy.

History—The patient may complain of a sudden onset of floaters, indicating pigment or blood in the vitreous, and flashing lights caused by traction on the retina. These, however, are not invariable and the patient may not present until there is field loss when the area of detachment is sufficiently large, or a deterioration in visual acuity if the macula is detached. Retinal detachment is more likely to occur if the retina is thin (in the shortsighted patient), damaged (by trauma), or if the ocular dynamics have been disturbed (by a previous cataract operation). Traction from contracting epiretinal scar tissue in a diabetic patient can also cause a retinal detachment.

Examination—The visual acuity is normal if the macula is still attached, but the acuity is reduced to counting fingers or hand movements if the macula is detached. Field loss (not complete in the early stages) is dependent on the size and location of the detachment. Direct ophthalmoscopy is not adequate to detect a retinal detachment if the detachment is small; detached retinal folds may be seen in larger detachments.

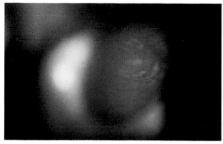

Small flat retinal hole encircled with laser burns.

Management—The patient should be referred urgently. Only small retinal holes with no associated fluid under the retina can be treated with the laser, which causes an inflammatory reaction that seals the hole. True detachments usually require an operation to seal any holes, reduce vitreous traction, and if necessary drain fluid from beneath the neuroretina.

Arterial occlusion

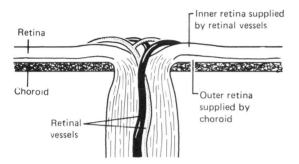

Blood supply of retina.

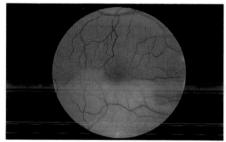

Infarction of lower half of retina.

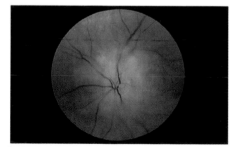

Ischaemic optic nerve head, pale and swollen.

History—The patient complains of a sudden onset of visual disturbance. This may be temporary (amaurosis fugax) if the obstruction dislodges, or it may be permanent. It is often described as a "curtain" descending over the vision.

Examination—The visual acuity depends on whether the macula or its fibres are affected. There may be no direct pupillary reaction if there is a complete occlusion of the central retinal artery. The extent of field loss depends on the area of the retina affected. The inner two thirds of the neuroretina is supplied by the retinal artery and its branches, and the outer third is supplied by the choroid. The arteries may be blocked by atherosclerosis, thrombosis, or emboli, and the attacks may be associated with a history of transient ischaemic attacks if the aetiology is embolic. When the retina infarcts it becomes oedematous and pale and masks the choroidal circulation except at the macula, which is extremely thin—hence the "cherry red spot" appearance. Ophthalmoscopy may be normal initially, before the oedema is established. As the oedema subsides the appearance returns to normal. Plaques of cholesterol or calcium may be seen in the vessels.

Management—Giant cell arteritis must be excluded by the history, examination, and performing an erythrocyte sedimentation rate. Emboli from the carotid arteries and the heart should also be excluded. Attempts may be made to open up the arterial circulation in acute cases by ocular massage, or by carbon dioxide rebreathing to cause arterial dilatation. Factors predisposing to vascular disease (for example, smoking, diabetes, and hyperlipidaemia) should be identified and treated.

Occlusion of the posterior ciliary arteries may cause ischaemia and infarction of the head of the optic nerve (ischaemic optic neuropathy). The nerve head swells and this may be mistaken for papilloedema. Papilloedema, however, is usually bilateral and the visual acuity is not affected until late in its development. In addition, the optic disc in ischaemic optic neuropathy is pale because of the lack of blood perfusion. Giant cell arteritis must be excluded in these cases as the other eye may also go blind if intravenous and oral steroid treatment is not started promptly.

Venous occlusion

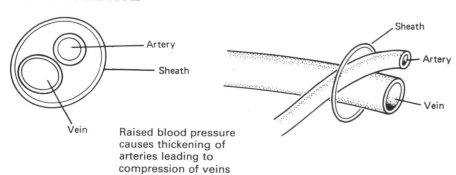

Raised blood pressure causes thickening of arteries leading to compression of veins

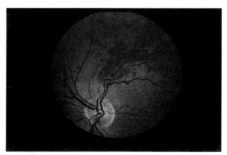

Branch retinal vein occlusion.

Acute visual disturbance

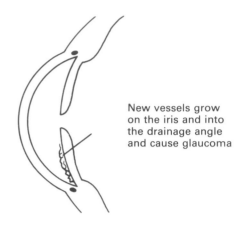

New vessels grow on the iris and into the drainage angle and cause glaucoma

Neovascularisation of the iris induced by vasoproliferative factors released from the ischaemic retina.

History—The visual acuity will be disturbed only if the occlusion affects the temporal arcades and damages the macula. Patients may otherwise complain only of a vague visual disturbance or of field loss. The arteries and veins share a common sheath in the eye, and venous occlusion most commonly occurs where arteries and veins cross, and in the head of the nerve. Thus raised arterial pressure can give rise to venous occlusion. Hyperviscosity—for example, in myeloma—and increased "stickiness" of the blood—as in diabetes mellitus—will also predispose to venous occlusion. This leads to haemorrhages and oedema of the retina. Occlusion of the central retinal vein within the head of the nerve leads to swelling of the optic disc.

Examination—Visual acuity will not be affected unless the macula is damaged. There may be only some peripheral field loss if a branch occlusion has occurred. Ophthalmoscopy shows characteristic flame haemorrhages in the affected areas, with a swollen disc if there is occlusion of the central vein. Cotton wool spots imply an ischaemic retina and are a bad prognostic sign.

Management—Hypertension, diabetes mellitus, hyperviscosity, and glaucoma must be identified and treated. If the retina becomes ischaemic it releases vasoproliferative factors which stimulate the formation of new vessels on the iris (rubeosis), and subsequent neovascularisation of the angle may lead to secondary glaucoma. Laser treatment is used to ablate the ischaemic retina to prevent this happening.

Disciform macular degeneration

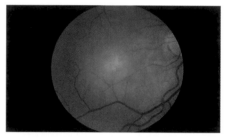

Leakage of fluid at macula.

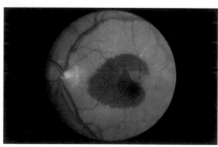

Macular haemorrhage.

History—The patient notices a sudden disturbance of central vision. Straight lines may seem wavy and objects may be distorted, even seeming larger or smaller than normal. Eventually central vision may be completely lost. This central area of visual distortion or loss moves as the patient attempts to look around it. The layer under the retina is the black retinal pigment epithelium. Most commonly with increasing age (the patient is normally over 60) and in certain conditions (for example, high myopia) neovascular membranes may develop under this layer in the macular region. These membranes may leak fluid or bleed causing an acute disturbance of vision.

Examination—The visual acuity depends on the extent of macular involvement. If the patient looks at a grid pattern (Amsler chart) the lines may look distorted centrally. The peripheral fields are normal. On fundal examination the macula may look normal, or there may be a raised area within it. Haemorrhage in the retina is red but it appears black if it is under the retinal pigment epithelium. There may be associated deposits of yellow degenerative retinal products (Drusen).

Management—Some cases are treatable with a laser, which occludes these neovascular membranes. If a patient has had a subretinal neovascular membrane in one eye that has destroyed central vision, they are at risk of the same thing occurring in the other eye.

Retrobulbar neuritis

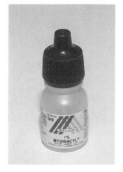
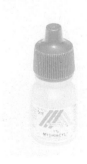

Red as seen by normal eye. Red desaturation.

History—The patient is usually a woman between the ages of 20 and 40 who complains of a disturbance of vision in one eye. There is usually pain that worsens on movement of the eye. The visual acuity may range from 6/6 to perception of light. Despite a "normal" visual acuity, however, the patient usually has an afferent pupillary defect and may also notice that the colour red looks faded when viewed with the affected eye (red desaturation). The field defect is usually located in the central field (central scotoma). It is extremely important to test the field of the other eye as a field defect may suggest a lesion further back (for example, a pituitary adenoma). The optic disc is swollen if the "inflammation" is anterior in the nerve. There may have been previous attacks in the past. If there are other symptoms of general demyelinating disease (such as pins and needles, weakness, or incontinence) these suggest disseminated sclerosis.

Management—Most patients recover spontaneously, but they may be left with diminished acuity and optic atrophy. Treatment with steroids does not alter the long term visual prognosis but may hasten the recovery. Treatment with high dose intravenous steroids has no significant effect on long term visual prognosis but may reduce the long term incidence of multiple sclerosis in selected patients. Referral to a neurologist is necessary. If there is doubt about the diagnosis the patient may need further investigation to exclude a space occupying lesion.

> **Treatment with steroids does not alter the visual prognosis, but may hasten recovery**

Migraine

History—Migraine may initially present with symptoms of visual loss. The features are well known and include:

- A family history of migraine
- Attacks set off by certain stimuli—for example, particular foods
- Fortification spectra in both eyes that include zig zag lines and multicoloured flashes of light
- Associated headaches and nausea (though these symptoms may not be present).

Examination—The patient may have a bilateral field defect but this usually resolves within a few hours.

Management—Conventional treatment with analgesics and antiemetics may be necessary. Long term prophylaxis may be required if attacks occur frequently.

> **Particular features**
> - Zigzag lines
> - Multicoloured flashing lights

Cardiovascular disease

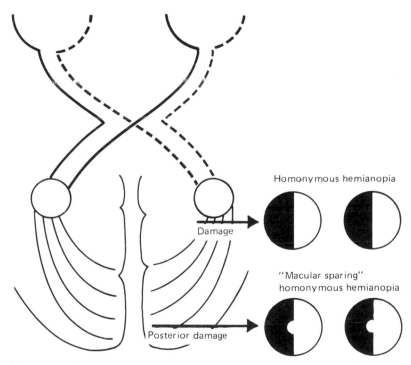

Damage to visual pathways leading to contralateral homonymous hemianopia

History—The patient may have a hemiparesis on the same side as the visual field loss. Patients sometimes complain of "the beginning or end of a line of print disappearing," and some may complain of a decrease in acuity. The visual pathways pass through a large area of the cerebral hemispheres, and any vascular occlusion in these areas will affect these pathways. Lesions behind the chiasm are the most common and lead to contralateral field loss in both eyes. More posteriorly placed lesions tend to spare the macular vision in the affected fields.

Examination—The visual acuity should be preserved though patients may say half the Snellen chart is missing. The appropriate bilateral visual field loss is present.

Management—It is important to make the diagnosis and exclude any underlying cause for vascular disease. The field defects sometimes improve with time, and patients should be taught to compensate for their field defect with appropriate head and eye movements.

CATARACTS

Symptoms

Difficulty in
• Reading
• Recognising faces
• Watching television
• Seeing in bright light
• Driving

"Cataract" is the term used to describe any lens opacity from the smallest dot to complete opacification. Cataracts are the most important cause of blindness in the world today. The prevalence of cataracts increases with age; 65% of people aged 50 to 59 have opacities and all of those aged over 80. Only when these opacities significantly interfere with vision is an operation contemplated.

Symptoms depend on whether the cataracts are unilateral or bilateral, and the degree and position of the opacity. If the cataract is unilateral the patient may not notice its effects until he has cause to cover the good eye. Patients may complain of difficulty in reading (which should be differentiated from the presbyopia that is normal in older people), in recognising faces, and in watching television. They may complain that their vision worsens in bright light, especially if the opacity is central. Occasionally patients experience monocular diplopia and see haloes round lights; this is due to the lens opacity interfering with light rays passing to the back of the eye. Some patients may even report that they can read without glasses. This happens when a nuclear sclerotic cataract increases the converging power of the lens, so making the patient myopic (short sighted).

Signs

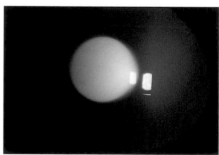

Pinhole

The signs of a cataract are:

A reduction in visual acuity—The degree of visual impairment depends on the nature of the cataract and the conditions of testing. Visual acuity should also be tested with a pin hole to eliminate refractive errors.

A diminished red reflex on ophthalmoscopy—When the ophthalmoscope is used to view the eye from about two feet away the reflection of the fundus can be seen as a "red reflex." This is the troublesome reflex so often seen in photographs of people taken with a flashlight. If there is any opacity between the cornea and the retina this reflex will have opacities in it. The nature of the opacities in the reflex will depend on the position and extent of the opacities in the optical media. This reflex is more easily seen when the pupil is dilated.

A change in the appearance of the lens—If one shines a bright light on the eye the lens may appear brown, or even white if the cataract is more advanced.

Although cataracts are common they are not the only cause of visual problems. The patient with a cataract should be able to point to the position of a light. Lack of normal "projection of light" should lead one to suspect problems either in the posterior part of the eye or beyond. The pupillary reactions should also be normal. If they are not, retinal disease or an abnormality of the visual pathway should be suspected.

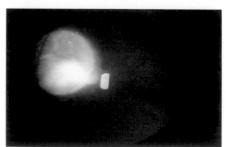

Clear red reflex.

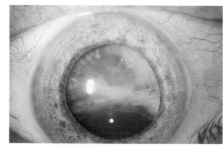

Opacities obscuring red reflex.

Cortical cataract.

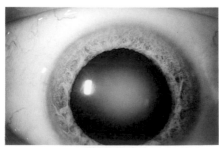

Nuclear sclerotic cataract.

Cataracts occurring in children are much more serious, as the development of vision may be irreversibly impaired (visual deprivation amblyopia) even if the cataracts are removed later. Any child with suspected cataracts should be referred immediately. Cataracts in young children are detected by looking at the red reflex, and this should be a routine part of the examination of a young child.

> **Children with cataracts must be referred immediately**

Causes

> - Age
> - Diabetes
> - Inflammation
> - Trauma
> - Steroids

There are many conditions that are associated with cataracts. Changes within the lens associated with aging are, however, the commonest cause of cataract. Cataracts also occur more often in patients with diabetes, uveitis, and a history of trauma to the eye. Prolonged courses of steroids, both oral and topical, can also give rise to cataracts. Children with cataracts need to be investigated to exclude treatable metabolic conditions such as galactosaemia.

Management

Extracapsular cataract surgery

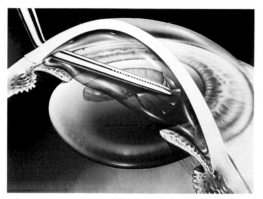

Removal of the anterior capsule of the lens.

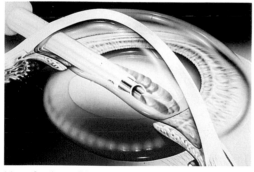

Liquefaction of lens nucleus with an ultrasonic probe.

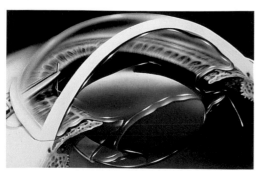

Plastic lens being inserted into the remaining clear capsular bag of the natural lens.

There is no effective medical treatment for established cataracts. The treatment is surgical.

Indications for operation

The decision to operate depends primarily on the effect of the cataracts on the patient's vision. With advances in operative techniques the operation may be done at any stage with minimal risk. There is no set level below which an operation is essential but most patients with vision of 6/18 or worse in both eyes as a result of lens opacities usually benefit from cataract extraction. Some elderly patients, however, may be perfectly happy with this level of vision. Simple advice may be adequate, such as recommending that they use a good reading light that provides illumination from above and behind.

A younger patient with more exacting visual demands may opt for operation much earlier. (The minimum standard for driving is about 6/10, which is equivalent to a line between 6/9 and 6/12.) With certain types of cataract, such as an opacity located at the back of the lens (posterior subcapsular cataract) the vision may be 6/6 in dim conditions when the pupil is dilated. In bright sunlight, however, the pupil constricts and most of the light that enters the eye has to pass through this opacity, which causes glare and a fall in acuity. If a patient found this disabling he or she could be operated on, even though the tested vision was 6/6. On the whole the surgeon's advice is tailored to the individual patient. The old concept of a "ripe" cataract is now obsolete. Most patients can be operated on under local anaesthesia as day cases.

Technique of operation

Extracapsular method—The anterior capsule is opened and the contents of the lens aspirated after the nucleus has been expressed. Years ago surgeons waited until the cataract was mature or "ripe" (when the contents became liquified) because this made aspiration of the lens easier. With advances in microsurgery, however, there is now no longer a need to wait for the cataract to mature. The extracapsular technique (where the clear capsular bag of the lens is left behind) is now the standard technique in developed countries. This operation can be done through a small incision (3 mm) as the nucleus can be liquified by an ultrasonic probe (phacoemulsification). This technological advance potentially improves the speed of recovery and visual rehabilitation after the operation.

Intracapsular method—The entire lens is removed within its capsule, usually with a cryoprobe, after the suspensory ligaments of the lens have been dissolved by the enzyme α-chymotrypsin. An iridectomy is done to stop the forward movement of the vitreous from blocking the flow of aqueous through the pupil. This method is now usually used only under special circumstances, or when a large number of cataract extractions have to be done without the insertion of lens implants.

Cataracts

Intracapsular cataract surgery

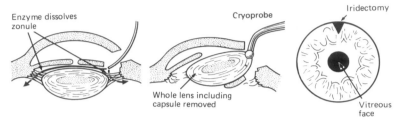

Enzyme dissolves zonule

Cryoprobe

Whole lens including capsule removed

Iridectomy

Vitreous face

Different types of lens implants.

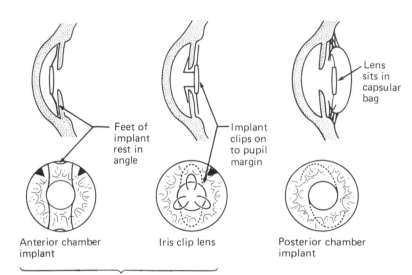

Feet of implant rest in angle

Implant clips on to pupil margin

Lens sits in capsular bag

Anterior chamber implant

Iris clip lens

Posterior chamber implant

Rarely used

Intraocular implants—An intraocular lens implant has the optical advantage of being placed in the eye like its natural counterpart, which overcomes the problems associated with spectacles and contact lenses. The final refractive state of the eye after operation can be chosen by taking into account the curvature of the cornea and the length of the eye (measured by ultrasonography) and then implanting a lens of appropriate power. Virtually all the lenses implanted nowadays are posterior chamber lenses, which are placed in the empty lens bag after the contents have been removed from the eye. With this type of lens the lens implant sits in its natural position and the pupil can be dilated without any problem. The other types of lenses (which are now rarely used) are anterior chamber lenses which are fixed in the angle of the anterior chamber of the eye, and the "pupil clip" lens which is clipped to the margin of the iris. The pupil should not be dilated if the "pupil clip" type has been used as the lens may dislocate.

- Steroid drops (inflammation)
- Antibiotic drops (infection)
- Dilating drops (adhesions)

Avoid strenuous exertion

Postoperative care

Most patients are treated for several weeks with steroid drops to reduce inflammation and antibiotic drops to prevent infection. Patients are traditionally advised to avoid activities that may raise the pressure in the eyeball appreciably, such as strenuous exercise or heavy lifting, for a few weeks after the operation.

If an extracapsular extraction has been done the remaining capsule may thicken (usually over a period of months or years) and this may require division. Thickening of the posterior capsule is the most common cause of progressive worsening of vision in patients who have had cataracts extracted. The thickened capsule is usually divided with a special laser that cuts tissue rather than burns it. This avoids the need to open the eye, and can be done in the outpatient department with the patient sitting at a slit-lamp microscope. This has contributed to the common misconception among patients that cataracts can be removed by laser.

Optical correction after operation

Removal of the lens results in an eye with a large hypermetropic (longsighted) refractive error for which the eye cannot compensate without artificial correction. This refractive error is now usually corrected with a plastic intraocular lens implant at the time of operation. If an implant has been inserted glasses will usually still be required for reading fine print as the new lens has a fixed focus. Intraocular lenses are available that allow two points of focus, but possible problems include reduced visual acuity and a reduction in perception of contrast so single focus intraocular lenses are normally used. If this is not possible for technical reasons, however, or the patient had had a previous cataract extraction before intraocular lenses were commonly used, optical correction can be achieved with a contact lens or spectacles.

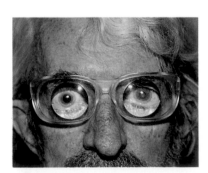

Cataract glasses: thick, heavy, expensive, with magnified image and reduced field of vision. Now rarely necessary because of intraocular lens implants.

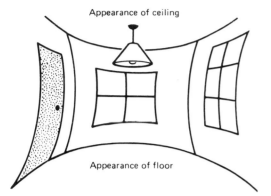

Appearance of ceiling

Appearance of floor

Peripheral image distortion that may be present with cataract spectacles.

Spectacles—The natural lens has great refractive power and consequently the spectacles required to correct the refractive error after cataract extraction are thick and heavy even when they are made of plastic. The corrected image is about 30% larger than that seen by the normal eye. This means that the image from an eye that has had a cataract extraction with subsequent spectacle correction cannot be fused with the other eye unless the cataract in the other eye is also removed. Objects are also perceived to be closer than they are, often resulting in accidents—for example, pouring tea into one's lap rather than into a cup. The field of vision is restricted and there is a "blind" area all round within this field because of the optical aberrations inherent in such powerful lenses. The effects of these problems can be minimised by the use of contact lenses or an intraocular lens implant.

Contact lenses—The size of an image with a contact lens is only 10% larger than the image in the normal eye. The brain can fuse this discrepancy so both an operated eye and an unoperated eye may be used simultaneously. Most patients, however, are elderly and problems may arise because of an inadequate tear film, difficulties with handling, and infection.

Secondary intraocular lens implantation—If the problems posed by using contact lenses or spectacles prove too much to overcome, secondary implantation of an intraocular lens can be considered. This is not without risk, however, particularly in eyes which have had previous intracapsular cataract extraction, and the potential advantages and disadvantages must be fully considered by the patient and the ophthalmologist before a decision is made.

REFRACTIVE ERRORS

The eye with no refractive error

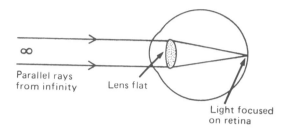

Parallel rays from infinity

Lens flat

Light focused on retina

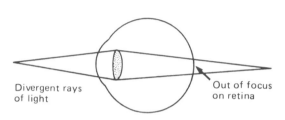

Divergent rays of light

Out of focus on retina

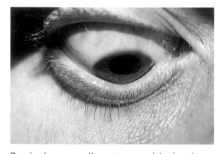

Conical cornea (keratoconus) indenting lower lid on down gaze.

Indistinct vision is most commonly caused by errors of refraction. Doctors do not often have to deal with this problem because patients are usually prescribed glasses by an optometrist. It is extremely important, however, to ask the question: "Is this patient's poor vision caused by a refractive error?"

The use of a simple "pinhole" made in a piece of card will help to determine whether there is a refractive error. In the absence of disease the vision will improve when the pinhole is used unless the refractive error is extremely large.

In an eye with no refractive error (emmetropia) light rays from infinity are brought to a focus on the retina by the cornea and lens when the eye is in a "relaxed" state. The cornea contributes about two thirds and the lens one third to the eye's refractive power. Disease affecting the cornea—for example, keratoconus—may cause severe refractive problems.

The rays of light from closer objects are divergent and have to be brought to a focus on the retina by the process of accommodation. The circular ciliary muscle contracts, allowing the naturally elastic lens to assume a more globular shape that has greater converging power. With age the lens gradually hardens and even when the ciliary muscle contracts the lens no longer becomes globular. Thus from the age of about 40 onwards close work becomes gradually more difficult (presbyopia). Objects may be held further away to reduce the need for accommodation, leading to the complaint "my arms don't seem to be long enough." At close range fine detail cannot be discerned.

No accommodation   **Accommodation**

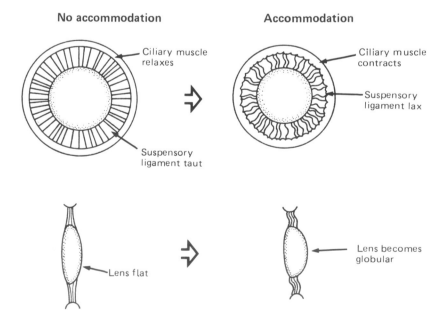

Ciliary muscle relaxes

Ciliary muscle contracts

Suspensory ligament lax

Suspensory ligament taut

Lens flat

Lens becomes globular

Convex lenses in the form of reading glasses are therefore needed to converge the light rays from close objects on to the retina. All emmetropic people need reading glasses for close work in later life. Eyes do not get worse if a person reads in bad light or does not wear his glasses; the exceptions are young children, who may need a refractive error corrected to prevent amblyopia.

The myopic or shortsighted eye

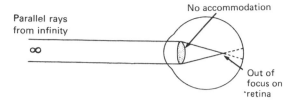

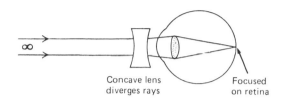

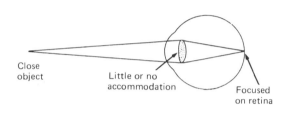

In the myopic eye light rays from infinity are brought to a focus in front of the retina either because the eye is too long or because the converging power of the cornea and lens is too great. To achieve clear vision the rays of light must be diverged by a concave lens so that light rays are focused on the retina.

For near vision light rays are focused on the retina with little or no accommodation depending on the degree of myopia and the distance at which the object is held—hence the fact that shortsighted people can often read without glasses even late in life, when those without refractive errors need reading glasses.

A certain type of cataract (nuclear sclerosis) increases the refractive power of the lens, making the eye more myopic. Patients with these cataracts may say that their reading vision has actually improved. Patients with an extreme degree of shortsightedness are more susceptible to retinal detachment, macular degeneration, and primary open angle glaucoma.

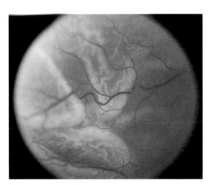

Retinal detachment.

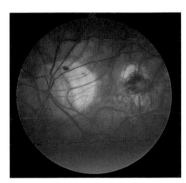

Macular degeneration with myopic crescent temporal to disc.

The hypermetropic or longsighted eye

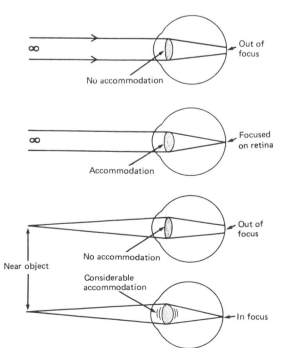

In the hypermetropic eye light rays from infinity are brought to a focus behind the retina either because the eye is too short or because the converging power of the cornea and lens is too weak. Unlike the young shortsighted person, the young longsighted person can achieve a clear retinal image by accommodating. Extremely good distance vision can often be achieved by this "fine tuning"—for example, 6/4 on the Snellen chart—and this has given rise to the term "longsighted."

For near vision the longsighted person has to accommodate even more. This may be possible during the first two or three decades of life, but the need for reading glasses arises earlier than in the normal person. Typically the longsighted person needs reading glasses at about 30 years of age. If a high degree of hypermetropia is present accommodation may not be adequate, and glasses may have to be worn for both distant and near vision from an earlier age.

As the ability to accommodate—and thus compensate for the hypermetropia—fails with the years, the longsighted person may require glasses for both distant and near vision when none were needed before. This may result in the complaint of a deterioration in eyesight because the patient has gone from not needing glasses to needing them for both distance and near vision.

Longsighted people are more susceptible to closed angle glaucoma because their shorter eyes are more likely to have shallow anterior chambers and narrow angles.

The astigmatic eye

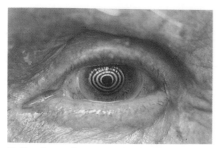

Reflections of concentric circles showing distortion by astigmatic cornea.

Astigmatism occurs when the cornea does not have an even curvature. A good analogy is that of a soccer ball (no astigmatism) and a rugby ball (astigmatism). The curvature of a normal cornea may be likened to that of the back of a ladle and that of the astigmatic eye to the back of a spoon. This uneven curvature results in an uneven focus in different meridians, and the eye cannot compensate by accommodating.

Astigmatism can be corrected by a lens that has power in only one meridian (a cylinder). Alternatively, an evenly curved surface may be achieved by fitting a hard contact lens. Astigmatism may be caused by any disease that affects the shape of the cornea—for example, a meibomian cyst may press hard enough on the cornea to cause distortion.

Contact lenses

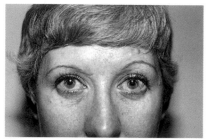

Gas permeable contact lenses to correct myopia.

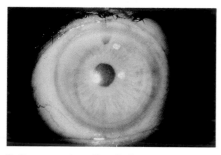

Soft contact lens fitted after cataract extraction

Contact lenses have become increasingly popular in recent years. There are several types, which can be grouped into three categories.

Hard lenses are made of polymethylmethacrylate and are not permeable to gases or liquids. They cannot be worn continuously because the cornea becomes hypoxic, and they are the most difficult lenses to get used to. Because of their rigidity, however, they correct astigmatism well and are durable. Infection and allergy are less likely with this type of lens. They are now less commonly prescribed, but there are still many people who have been using them for a long time with no problems.

Gas permeable lenses have properties between hard and soft lenses. They allow the passage of oxygen through to the tear film and the cornea, and they are better tolerated than hard lenses. Being semirigid they correct astigmatism better than soft lenses. They are, however, more prone to the accumulation of deposits and are less durable than hard lenses. Gas permeable lenses are usually used as daily wear lenses.

Soft lenses have a high water content and are permeable to both gases and liquids. They are tolerated much better than hard or gas permeable lenses and may be worn for longer periods. Both infection and allergy, however, are more common. The lenses are also less durable, are more prone to the accumulation of deposits, and do not correct astigmatism as do the harder lenses. Nevertheless, because they are so well tolerated they are now the most commonly prescribed lenses.

Certain types of gas permeable and soft lenses can be worn continuously for up to several months because of their high oxygen permeability, but the risk of sight threatening complications is significantly higher than with daily wear lenses.

Disposable lenses are soft lenses that are designed to be thrown away after a period of continuous use. They are popular because no cleaning is required during this period. However, the lenses must be disposed of as recommended, or the risk of complications such as corneal infection rises significantly.

Indications for prescribing contact lenses

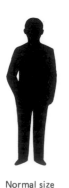
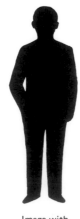
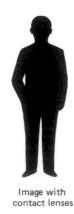
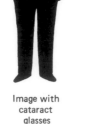

Normal size image

Image with cataract glasses

Image with contact lenses

Personal appearance and the inconvenience of spectacles are common reasons for prescribing contact lenses. They may also considerably reduce the optical aberrations that are associated with the wearing of glasses, particularly those with high power such as are sometimes prescribed for patients who have undergone cataract extraction. The brain cannot resolve the large difference in the size of the retinal images that occurs when the refractive power of the two eyes differs considerably. A good example of this is if a cataract has been removed from only one eye and a spectacle lens has been prescribed, whilst the other eye is normal. A contact lens brings the image size closer to "normal," permitting the brain to fuse the two images. A contact lens permits irregularities in the cornea to be neutralised, and the effects of an irregularly shaped cornea—for example, keratoconus—may by corrected. If a patient is very myopic, contact lenses may increase the size of the image and improve the visual acuity.

Relative contraindications to wearing contact lenses

- Atopy
- Dry eyes
- Inability to handle lenses

Contraindications include a history of atopy, "dry eyes" and an inability to handle or cope with the management of lenses. These are, however, relative contraindications; a trial of lenses may be the only way to determine whether it is feasible for a particular patient to wear contact lenses.

Complications of wearing contact lenses

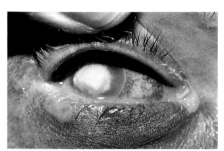

Corneal abscess associated with contact lens wear.

The most serious complication of contact lens wear is a corneal abscess. This is most common in elderly patients who have worn soft contact lenses for an extended period. Corneal abrasions are fairly common. Any contact lens wearer with a red eye should have the lens removed and the eye stained with fluorescein to show up any corneal abrasion or abscess. **Because fluorescein stains soft contact lenses the eye should be washed out with saline before the lens is replaced.** If there is an abrasion or infection the appropriate treatment should be given, and the contact lens *should not be worn again* until the condition has resolved.

The wearing time may have to be built up again, particularly if hard or gas-permeable lenses are worn. Good hygiene is essential for wearers of contact lenses to minimise the risks of infection. Lenses should never be licked and placed back in the eye. A booklet of guidelines for the patients outlining risks, proper care of lenses, and action to be taken if problems arise has been published by the Department of Health and this (or a similar one) should be given to patients who are being fitted with contact lenses.

Refractive surgery

Myopic (short sighted eye)

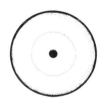

Light rays focus in front of retina

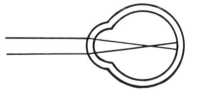

Radial keratotomy
Cuts made in the periphery of the cornea

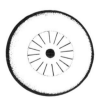

Peripheral cornea steepens and central cornea flattens focusing light on retina

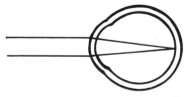

Photorefractive keratectomy
Central cornea reshaped by laser

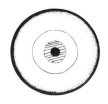

Central cornea flattened focusing light on retina

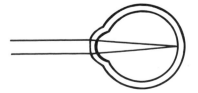

There has been much interest in operations to alter the refractive state of the eye, particularly to treat myopia and any associated astigmatism. The technique called radial keratotomy entails making deep radial incisions in the peripheral cornea which result in flattening of the central cornea and refocusing of light rays nearer the retina. It is of use only in myopia and possible disadvantages include weakening of the cornea (particularly if the eye is injured subsequently), infection, glare, and diurnal fluctuation of the refractive state of the eye. If contact lenses are still required after radial keratotomy they are much more difficult to fit.

More recently a special laser (excimer laser) has been used to reshape the surface of the cornea. This works by vapourising a thin layer of the cornea (photoablation), which alters the curve of the front surface of the cornea and changes its focusing power. This technique is theoretically safer than radial keratotomy as it does not involve deep cuts into the eye. Side effects include pain for a few days after the laser treatment, a period during which the eye is overcorrected and becomes longsighted, opacification of the treated zone (which may result in a—usually transient—reduction of best corrected visual acuity), and poor predictability of the final refractive result if the patient is extremely shortsighted. Contraindications to excimer laser corneal surgery include autoimmune disease, and previous herpes simplex infection of the cornea which may be reactivated. If patients are contemplating any kind of refractive surgery it is important that they are fully informed of the risks by the operating surgeon and have time to evaluate the advantages and disadvantages before undergoing a procedure that may cause irreversible change.

THE GLAUCOMAS

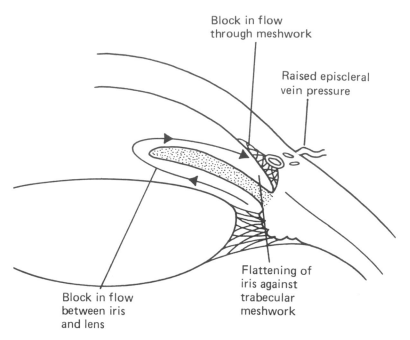

Block in flow
through meshwork

Raised episcleral
vein pressure

Block in flow
between iris
and lens

Flattening of
iris against
trabecular
meshwork

Normal aqueous drainage and possible sites of obstruction.

The glaucomas are a range of disorders that are characterised by optic disc cupping, visual field loss, and an intraocular pressure sufficiently raised to damage the eye. This group of disorders is the third most common cause of blindness world wide.

Normally the ciliary body secretes aqueous, which then flows through the posterior chamber and through the pupil into the anterior chamber. It then leaves the eye through the trabecular meshwork, flowing into the canal of Schlemm and into episcleral veins. The flow and drainage can be obstructed in several ways (See diagram).

- **The clinical signs of raised intraocular pressure depend on both the rate and degree of the rise in pressure**

Symptoms and signs

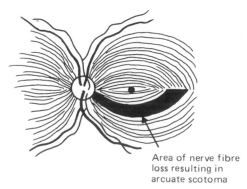

Cloudy cornea after sudden rise in intraocular pressure (acute angle closure glaucoma).

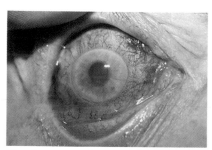

Area of nerve fibre loss resulting in arcuate scotoma

Normal distribution of nerve fibres in the retina.

The patient with primary open angle glaucoma (also known as chronic open angle glaucoma) may not notice any symptoms until severe visual damage has occurred. This is because the rise in pressure and consequent damage occur so slowly that the patient has time to compensate. In contrast, the clinical presentation of acute closed angle glaucoma is well known as the intraocular pressure rises rapidly and results in a red, painful eye with disturbance of vision.

Haloes around lights and a cloudy cornea—The cornea is kept transparent by the continuous removal of fluid by the endothelial cells. If the pressure rises slowly this process takes longer to fail. When the pressure rises quickly (acute closed angle glaucoma) the cornea becomes waterlogged, causing a fall in visual acuity and giving rise to the symptom of haloes (analogous to looking at a light through frosted glass).

Pain—If the rise in pressure is slow, pain is not a feature of glaucoma until the pressure is extremely high. Pain is not a feature of primary open angle glaucoma.

Field loss—The normal distribution of the retinal nerve fibres is shown. Pressure on the nerve fibres and chronic ischaemia at the head of the nerve cause damage to these fibres and usually result in a characteristic pattern of field loss (arcuate scotoma). This, however, spares central vision initially, and the patient may not notice the defect. Sophisticated techniques are required to detect early visual field defects. The terminal stage of glaucomatous field loss is a field that is severely contracted with only a few remaining fibres from the more richly innervated macular area surviving. Even at this stage (tunnel vision) the vision may still be 6/6 despite virtually no visual field remaining.

Disc changes—The optic disc marks the exit point of the retinal nerve fibres from the eye. In the presence of a sustained rise in pressure the nerve fibres atrophy, leaving the characteristic cupped disc of chronic glaucoma.

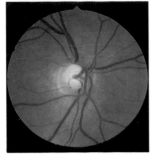

Glaucomatous cupping of optic disc.

Venous occlusion—Raised intraocular pressure can impede blood flow in the low pressure venous system predisposing to venous occlusion.

Enlargement of the eye—In the adult no enlargement of the eye is possible because growth has ceased. In a young child, however, the eye may expand causing enlargement of the eye (buphthalmos or "ox eye"). These children may also be photophobic, have a watering eye, and cloudy corneas.

Primary open angle glaucoma

Groups at risk:

- Older age groups
- Relatives of patients
- Diabetics
- Extremely shortsighted patients

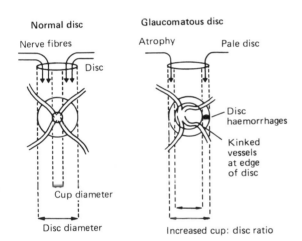

Optic disc changes in glaucoma.

Primary open angle glaucoma is the commonest form of glaucoma and is the third most common cause of blind registration in the United Kingdom. The resistance to outflow through the trabecular meshwork gradually increases for reasons that are not fully understood, and the pressure in the eye slowly increases causing damage to the nerve. The level of intraocular pressure is the main risk factor for visual loss. There may also be other mechanisms of damage, particularly ischaemia of the optic nerve head.

Symptoms—Because the visual loss is gradual patients do not usually present until severe damage has occurred. The disease can be detected by screening high risk groups for the signs of glaucoma. At present most patients with primary open angle glaucoma are detected by optometrists at routine examinations.

Groups at risk—The prevalence increases with age from 0·02% in the 40–49 age group to 10% in those aged over 80. First degree relatives of patients are at risk (one in 10), as are diabetics and extremely shortsighted people. People of Afro-Caribbean origin are also at increased risk.

Signs—The eye is white and quiet. Field loss is difficult to pick up clinically until considerable damage has occurred. The best signs for the purpose of detection are the disc changes. The cup:disc ratio increases as the nerve fibres atrophy. Asymmetry of disc cupping is also important, as the disease is often more advanced in one eye than the other. Haemorrhages on the optic disc are a poor prognostic sign.

Acute angle closure glaucoma

Groups at risk:

- Older patients
- Longsighted patients

Acute angle closure glaucoma is probably the best known type of glaucoma as the presentation is acute and the affected eye becomes red and painful. In angle closure glaucoma apposition of the lens to the back of the iris prevents the flow of aqueous from the posterior

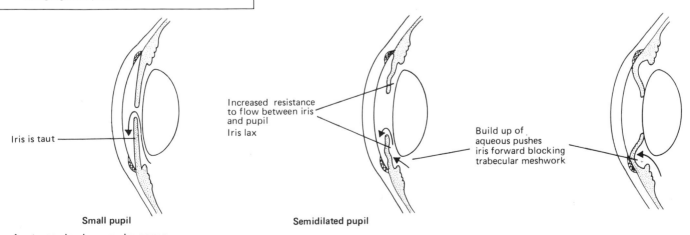

Acute angle closure glaucoma.

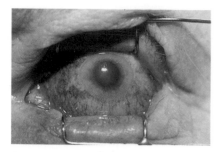

Acute angle closure glaucoma.

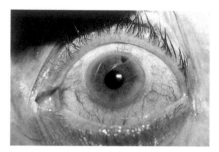

Surgical peripheral iridectomy.

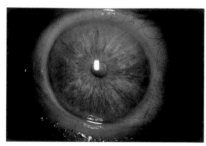

Laser iridotomies.

chamber to the anterior chamber. This is more likely to occur when the pupil is semidilated in the dark. Aqueous then collects behind the iris and pushes it on to the trabecular meshwork preventing the drainage of aqueous from the eye, and the intraocular pressure raises rapidly.

Symptoms—The eye becomes red and painful because of the rapid rise in intraocular pressure, and this is often associated with vomiting. Vision is blurred because the cornea becomes oedematous and patients may notice haloes around lights because of the dispersion of light. They may give a history of similar attacks in the past that were aborted by going to sleep. During sleep the pupil constricts and may pull the peripheral iris out of the angle.

Groups at risk—This type of glaucoma usually occurs in longsighted people, whose anterior chambers are shallow, and in the elderly, in whom the lens is larger. Acute angle closure glaucoma is more common in women than men.

Signs—The visual acuity is impaired depending on the degree of corneal oedema. The eye is red and tender to touch. The cornea is hazy because of oedema, and the pupil is semidilated and fixed to light. The attack begins with the pupil in the semidilated position and the rise in pressure makes the iris ischaemic and fixed in that position. On gentle palpation the affected eye feels much harder than the other. If the patient is seen shortly after an attack has resolved none of these signs may be present, hence the importance of the history.

Management—Emergency treatment is required if the sight of the eye is to be preserved. If it is not possible to get the patient to hospital straight away, acetazolamide (Diamox) 500 mg should be given intravenously, and pilocarpine 4% instiled in the eye to constrict the pupil. The intraocular pressure must first be brought down medically, and a hole must subsequently be made in the iris either surgically or with the laser in order to restore normal aqueous flow. The other eye should be similarly treated as a prophylactic measure. If the treatment is delayed adhesions may form between the iris and the cornea (peripheral anterior synechiae) and the trabecular meshwork may be damaged. A surgical drainage procedure may then be required.

Other types of glaucoma

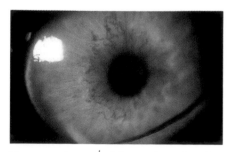

New vessels on the iris causing rubeotic glaucoma.

- Topical steroids may cause a change in the drainage meshwork resulting in a slow rise in intraocular pressure
- Patients may not complain of visual symptoms until severe damage has occurred

If there is inflammation in the eye (anterior uveitis) adhesions may develop between the lens and the iris (posterior synechiae). These adhesions will block the flow of the aqueous between the posterior and anterior chambers and result in forward ballooning of the iris and a rise in the intraocular pressure. Adhesions may also develop between the iris and the cornea (peripheral anterior synechiae) covering up the trabecular meshwork drainage area. Inflammatory cells may also block up the meshwork. Topical steroids may cause a gradual asymptomatic rise in intraocular pressure which may lead to blindness. Patients taking topical steroids long term should always be under ophthalmological supervision.

The growth of new vessels on to the iris (rubeosis) occurs both in diabetics and after occlusion of the central retinal vein as a consequence of retinal ischaemia. These vessels also block the trabecular meshwork, causing rubeotic glaucoma, which is extremely difficult to treat.

The trabecular meshwork itself may have developed abnormally (congenital glaucoma) or been damaged by trauma to the eye. Patients who have had eye injuries have a higher chance than normal of developing glaucoma later in life. If there is a bleed in the eye after trauma the red cells may also block the trabecular meshwork.

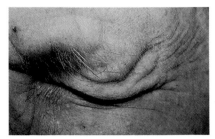

Eye closure after instilling drops to reduce systemic side effects.

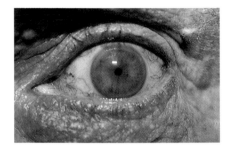

Small pupil with pilocarpine drops.

Topical treatment—β blockers—for example, timolol—reduce the secretion of aqueous and are the topical treatment of choice. Contraindications to their use include a history of lung or heart disease, as the drops may cause systemic β blockade. Systemic effects can be reduced by occlusion of the punctum or shutting the eyes for several minutes after putting in the drops, which stops the drops running down the lacrimal passages and being absorbed systemically through the nasal nasal mucosa or by inhalation directly into the lungs.

Parasympathomimetic agents—for example, pilocarpine—constrict the pupil and "pull" on the trabecular meshwork, increasing the flow of aqueous out of the eye. The small pupil may, however, cause visual problems if central lens opacities are present. Constriction of the ciliary body may cause accommodation and blurred vision particularly in young patients. Pilocarpine should not be used if there is inflammation in the eye as the pupil may stick to the lens close to the visual axis (posterior synechiae) and affect the vision.

Sympathomimetic agents—for example, adrenaline—may also be used. They increase the outflow of aqueous from the eye but dilate the pupil. They should not be used in eyes with shallow anterior chambers as closed angle glaucoma may be precipitated by dilatation of the pupil. Adrenaline causes local irritation and may have cardiovascular side effects due to systemic absorption. These side effects can be reduced by using a pro-drug that converts to its active form only when in the eye. Adrenaline has a minimal effect on intraocular pressure when a β blocker is already being used.

Oral or intravenous treatment—Carbonic anhydrase inhibitors—for example, acetazolamide—reduce the secretion of aqueous and are the most powerful drugs for reducing intraocular pressure. Unfortunately they have many side effects, including nausea, lassitude, parasthesiae, and renal stones.

Laser treatment

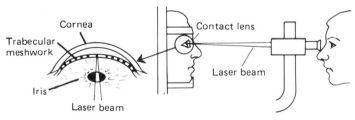

Laser trabeculoplasty.

Laser trabeculoplasty—Argon laser "burns" are applied to the trabecular meshwork. This may work by contracting one part of the meshwork, so stretching and opening up adjacent areas, but more recently it has been postulated that it rejuvenates the cells in the trabecular meshwork. This treatment is used only in the types of glaucoma in which the drainage angle is open. The pressure lowering effects are relatively short term, so this treatment is used mainly for more elderly patients.

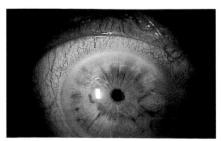

Hole made in the iris (iridotomy) with the neodymium YAG laser without having to cut into the eyeball.

Laser iridotomy can be performed in cases of angle closure glaucoma with the neodymium YAG laser, which—unlike the argon laser—actually cuts holes in tissue rather than just burning. This procedure can be performed without opening the eye surgically.

Surgical treatment

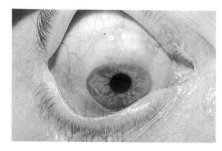

Conjunctival bleb after drainage operation.

Iridectomy is performed in cases of angle closure glaucoma both in the affected eye and prophylactically in the other eye, but most of the cases previously treated in this way can be treated with the neodymium YAG laser.

Drainage operation—A channel is created between the inside of the eye and the subconjunctival space, thus bypassing the blocked trabecular meshwork. A drainage "bleb" can often be seen under the upper lid. Conjunctivitis in a patient with a drainage bleb should always be treated promptly as there is an increased risk of the infection entering the eye (endophthalmitis). Surgery was previously undertaken only when medical treatment had failed to halt the progress of the disease. It is now being done much earlier as it lowers intraocular pressure more effectively than medical or laser treatments. The main cause of failure is scarring, but this can be controlled in most cases by short single treatments with drugs that reduce scarring. There is an increased incidence of cataracts after drainage operations.

Support group

The International Glaucoma Association is the major support group for patients with glaucoma in the United Kingdom. This organisation provides information and support for people with different forms of glaucoma.

International Glaucoma Association
Kings College Hospital
Denmark Hill
London SE5 9RS

Tel/Fax 0171 737 3265

GRADUAL VISUAL LOSS, PARTIAL SIGHT, AND "BLINDNESS"

Causes of gradual visual loss

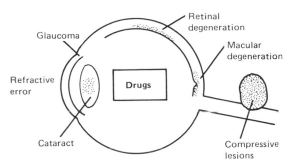

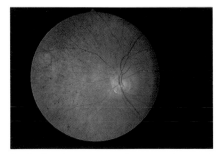

Cataract.

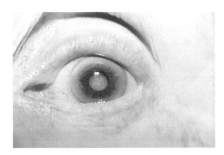

Retinitis pigmentosa:pigmentation and attenuated vessels.

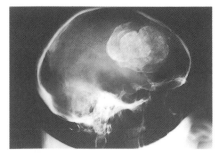

Radiograph showing calcified meningioma. Note a plain skull radiograph will not show most intracranial tumours.

● *Refractive error*—The pinhole test is a most useful test for identifying refractive error. If there is a refractive error the vision will improve. If the patient has strong glasses the pinhole should be used with the patient wearing the glasses. Once other causes of visual loss have been excluded, the patient can be sent to the optometrist for refraction.

● *Cataract*—This is probably the commonest cause of gradual visual loss and the diagnosis may be made on viewing the red reflex. The patient should be referred if the visual disturbance interferes appreciably with his lifestyle. If a patient with a cataract cannot project light or has an afferent pupillary defect, however, other diseases must be excluded.

● *Primary open angle glaucoma*—Unfortunately the patient may not complain of visual disturbance until late in the course of the disease, hence the need for screening. Primary open angle glaucoma should, however, be excluded in any patient complaining of gradual visual loss. Any family history of glaucoma should be elicited. The vision may still be 6/6 so the visual field should be checked with a red pin, and cupping of or asymmetry between the optic discs should be sought.

● *Age related macular degeneration*—This may occur gradually and is characterised by loss of the central field. There are usually pigmentary changes at the macula. The disease occurs in both eyes, but it may be asymmetrical, and it is more common in short sighted patients. The gradual deterioration is not treatable, but if acute visual distortion supervenes during the course of the disease there may be a leaking area under the retina that may be treated with the laser.

● *Hereditary degeneration of the retina*—This is relatively rare but should be suspected if there is a family history of visual deterioration. Symptoms include night blindness and intolerance to light. Most types of degeneration are not treatable, but some are associated with metabolic disorders and the visual deterioration may be arrested by treatment of the metabolic abnormality. These patients need to be referred for diagnosis, treatment, discussion of prognosis, and genetic counselling and to be informed about social services and voluntary organisations.

● *Compressive lesions of the optic pathways*—These are relatively rare, but should always be considered. The history and examination may give clues if there are headaches, focal neurological signs, or endocrinological abnormalities such as acromegaly. There should not be an afferent pupillary defect in most patients with cataract, macular degeneration, or refractive error. Testing of visual fields may show the bitemporal defect of a pituitary tumour. The discs should be checked for optic atrophy and papilloedema.

● *Drugs*—Several drugs may cause visual loss. In particular, a history of excessive alcohol intake or smoking, methanol ingestion, or the taking of chloroquine or ethambutol should lead to a suspicion of drug induced visual deterioration. Systemic steroids may cause cataracts and steroid drops may induce glaucoma.

Management of gradual visual loss

- Strong light from behind
- Magnifying aids
- Large print books
- Closed circuit television

Useful publications

Talking books:
Calibre
Aylesbury, Buckinghamshire HP22 5XQ. Tel 0296 432339.
Postal service of talking books on normal cassettes for registered blind and partially sighted people.

Royal London Society for the Blind
(address on page 41).
Books recorded on normal cassettes—postal service for registered blind and partially sighted people.

RNIB Talking Book Service
Mount Pleasant, Wembley, Middlesex HA0 1RR. Tel 081 903 6666.
Special machine with simple controls supplied.

Talking Newspaper Association of the UK
90 High Street, Heathfield, East Sussex TN21 8JO. Tel 0435 866102.
Registered charity that aims to make a taped newspaper available to every visually handicapped person in the country. Send a stamped addressed envelope for details.

Large print books:
Chivers Press Publishers, Windsor Bridge Road, Bath, Avon BA2 3AX.
Isis, 55 St Thomas's Street, Oxford OX1 1JG. Tel 0865 250333.
Magna, Magna House, Long Preston, Nr Skipton, North Yorkshire BC23 4ND. Tel 0729 840225.
Ulverscroft, The Green, Bradgate Road, Anstey, Leicester LE7 7FU. Tel 0533 364325.
  For a more comprehensive list see the *In touch* handbook (below), and the *Guide to UK Organisations for visually disabled people* (published by the RNIB).

Publications and programmes:
The *In touch* handbook is the most comprehensive publication available. It is published yearly and available in print, braille, and on tape. Transcription is available on request from the RNIB. Obtainable from BBC Broadcasting Support Services, PO Box 7, London W3 6XJ.
  A Radio 4 programme (called *In touch*) every Tuesday evening reports on developments that affect the daily lives of the million or more people in Britain who have a visual handicap.

Department of Social Security, Leaflets Unit, PO Box 21, Stanmore, Middlesex HA7 1AY. Tel 081 972 2000. Supplies patient leaflets about benefits.

Help starts here, a guide for parents of children with special needs including visual disability is published by the National Children's Bureau on behalf of the Council for Disabled Children, 8 Wakley Street, London EC1V 7QE.
Tel 071 278 9441.

The initial management of gradual visual loss depends on the cause. Refractive errors usually require no more than a pair of glasses. Cataracts can be removed and an artificial lens implanted. Glaucoma requires treatment to lower the intraocular pressure. There are, however, a large number of conditions that are not amenable to medical or surgical treatment. Despite this, there is still much that can be done for the patient.

- *Good lighting*—The patient should be advised to use adequate lighting. Using a stronger light bulb may make all the difference. Patients should be advised to read with a strong light placed behind them. A booklet called *Lighting and low vision* is available from the Partially Sighted Society.

- *Low vision aids*—A simple magnifying glass may be a great help. Books with large print are available from most public libraries. There are also special magnifying aids that can be attached to glasses; these differ from a simple magnifying glass in that they allow magnification without the patient having to get extremely close to the print. Many eye hospitals have a low vision aids service that is usually run by an optometrist. It may be possible to obtain such aids on loan from these departments. Closed circuit television can be used to magnify text and may allow a visually handicapped person to do a normal job. Various home aids are also available, such as braille knobs for cookers. Details are available from the Royal National Institute for the Blind (RNIB).

- *Registration as partially sighted or blind*—This confers various benefits, which are shown below. The patient has to be referred to a consultant ophthalmologist who completes a form (BD8). The requirements for registration are:
Partially sighted—The patient must have vision of 6/60 or worse in both eyes. The vision can be better than 6/60 if the visual fields are appreciably reduced—for example, a patient with 6/6 vision but severely restricted fields caused by primary open angle glaucoma.
Blind—The current statutory definition of blindness is "that a person should be so blind as to be unable to perform any work for which eyesight is essential." The guidelines for registration as blind are a visual acuity of 3/60 or worse in both eyes. Again, the visual acuity may be better than this if the visual fields are impaired.
  These criteria are flexible and the final decision is left to the consultant ophthalmologist who will take other ocular problems into consideration. It is important that the patient does not feel that all hope is lost and eventually everything will go "dark." This is particularly the case for patients with age related macular degeneration where only central vision is lost. In this case the patient can be told that he will not go blind because he will still have peripheral vision. A patient with a visual acuity of only counting fingers may still be virtually independent within the home despite being registered as blind.

Registration is necessary to qualify for financial benefits. It is not required, but is helpful, when initiating specialist support and advice from local authorities. A register of blind and partially sighted people living within the area is kept by each Department of Social Services. The social worker is the key person to contact, but a visually handicapped person may need a range of support services.

- *Mobility and technical training*—Mobility officers for the blind, who can be contacted through the social services, give mobility training for the visually handicapped. A technical officer is trained to teach communication and skills of daily living. Often technical and mobility skills are taught by a rehabilitation officer. Guide dogs for the blind are available in certain circumstances from the Guide Dogs for the Blind Association, a voluntary organisation.

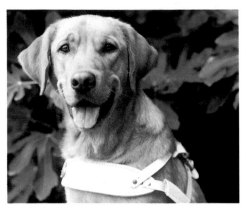
Guide dog.

- *Employment and training*—Information and advice are available from the RNIB Employment Network and from local job centres (Department of Employment).
- *Special education and training*—Advice about mainstream and special schools for visually handicapped children can be obtained from local education authorities. Help and advice for parents, particularly about their child's placement and their right of appeal, is offered by the RNIB advocatory service for parents. The policy of teaching visually handicapped children in normal schools depends on the local education authority. There are, however, special schools for severely disabled children where their particular needs are taken into account and specialised equipment and teaching are available. Training in work skills are available at various centres, details of which can be obtained from the RNIB.
- *Self help support groups and other organisations*—Apart from the RNIB there is a weekly radio programme called *In touch* for the visually handicapped. There is also the *In touch bulletin* which is in braille and available free from the BBC. The BBC also publishes a comprehensive guide to aids and services for the blind. Parents often ask to have contact with other parents to enable them to meet and share experiences at a time of crisis. There is a list of such groups in the *In touch* handbook.

Useful addresses and telephone numbers

Specifically for the visually handicapped:

Royal National Institute for the Blind (RNIB)
224 Great Portland Street, London W1N 6AA.
Tel 071 388 1266.
Benefits rights, community education, education and leisure, employment network, grants information, health services consultancy, information service on multiple disability, and many other services (see the *In touch* handbook).

Partially Sighted Society (registered office)
Queen's Road, Doncaster DN1 2NX. Tel 0302 323132. Greater London Office, 62 Salisbury Road, London NW6 6RU.
Tel 071 372 1551.
Over 20 local self help branches, provision of equipment and advice on living and working with impaired vision.

Guide Dogs for the Blind Association
Hillfields, Burghfield Common, Reading, Berkshire RG7 3YG.
Tel 0734 835555.
Offers a range of services to owners of guide dogs, applicants, and people considering application.

Action for Blind People (head office)
14/16 Verney Road, London SE16 3DZ. Tel 071 289 6111.
Offers information and advice about all available services for blind and partially sighted people including benefits and grants.

North Regional Association for the Blind
Headingley Castle, Headingley Lane, Leeds, West Yorkshire LS6 2DQ. Tel 0532 75266/7.

Royal London Society for the Blind (RLSB) (head office)
105 Salisbury Road, London NW6 6RH. Tel 071 624 8844
Runs sheltered workshops specialising in engineering contract work. Sponsorship for sheltered placement scheme and homeworker schemes. Education and further education college.

Southern Regional Association for the Blind
55 Eton Avenue, London NW3 3ET. Tel 071 722 9703.

SENSE (National Society for Deaf/Blind and Rubella Handicapped)
11-13 Clifton Terrace, Finsbury Park, London N4 3SR.
Tel 071 272 7774.
Campaigns for needs of deaf/blind children and young adults, and provides advice, support, information, and services for them, their families, and professionals.

General:
Age concern (England)
Astral House, 1268 London Road, Stanmore, Middlesex HA7 1AY. Tel 081 679 8000.
Provides insurance, day care centres, legal advice, home helps, and many other services.

Disabled Living Foundation
380–4 Harrow Road, London W9 2HU. Tel 071 289 6111.
Information about equipment for daily living for disabled people. Primarily a subscription service for professionals. Has an equipment centre open to the public but please telephone for an appointment.

The Family Fund
Joseph Rowntree Foundation, PO Box 50, York YO1 2XZ. Tel 0904 621115.
Helps families of severely handicapped children.

National Association of Toy and Leisure Libraries Association
68 Churchway, London NW1 1LT. Tel 071-387-9592.
Does not stock toys but provides details of local toy libraries.

Resource Centres
In most areas there are specialist centres where blind or partially sighted people can obtain information and advice. The range of equipment on display varies from one centre to another.

SQUINT

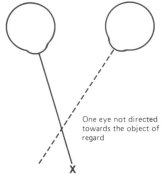

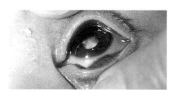

One eye not directed towards the object of regard

The subject of squint (strabismus) is one that many practitioners approach with great trepidation, sometimes with justification. If, however, it is approached systematically much of the myth and mystery can be dispelled.

What is a squint? The word is used in many different ways. It is often used to describe the narrowing of the gap between the upper and lower eyelids (interpalpebral fissure), usually by patients, creating a pinhole effect. This reduces the consequences of any refractive error and improves the clarity of the image. The true definition of squint, however, is that one of the eyes is not directed towards the object under scrutiny. It should be noted that when the eyes converge for close work there is no squint.

Why is a squint important?

Congenital cataract.

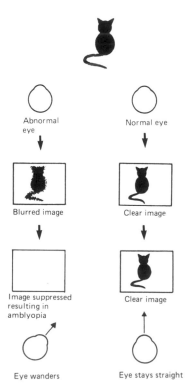

A squint may be a sign of impaired visual acuity.

● *A squint may show that the acuity of the eye is impaired* because of ocular disease. The eyes are kept straight by the drive to keep the image of the object being viewed in the centre of the macular area where highest definition and colour vision are located. The tone in the extraocular muscles is constantly being readjusted to maintain this fixation. If the vision is impaired in one or both eyes this constant readjustment cannot occur and one eye may wander. This is important, as the cause of impaired vision may be eminently treatable, as in the case of a cataract or a refractive error. It is especially important in a child because—unlike an adult—a child's vision may be irreversibly impaired if treatment is not given in time. The visual pathways in the brain receiving information from an abnormal eye fail to develop normally. The resulting depressed cortical function leads to amblyopia or a "lazy" eye. It is important to realise that a child does not complain that the sight of one eye is poor, and the prevention of permanent visual impairment in a child's eye may require no more than a pair of glasses to correct a refractive error.

● *The squint may itself cause amblyopia in a child*—Misalignment of the eyes may be the primary problem, with resulting double vision. In a young child the vision of one eye may be suppressed to avoid this diplopia and the visual pathways then fail to develop properly. This leads to amblyopia in an eye that is otherwise organically sound.

● *A squint may be a sign of a life threatening condition*—Squint is a common presentation in a child with a retinoblastoma. The resulting squint is non-paralytic and therefore the angle of deviation is the same irrespective of the direction of the gaze. The eye deviates because vision is impaired and this may occur in any eye with visual impairment. A squint may also be caused by a sixth nerve palsy resulting from a

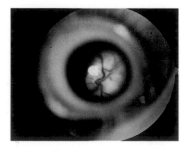

Retinoblastoma in a child presenting with a squint.

Patients with myasthenia gravis may present with squint and diplopia.

tumour that is causing raised intracranial pressure. In this case the squint will be paralytic and the angle of squint will vary depending on the direction of gaze. Patients with myasthenia gravis may first present with squint and diplopia.

How can a squint be detected and assessed clinically?

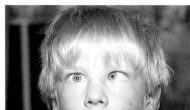

Left convergent squint: note position of light reflexes.

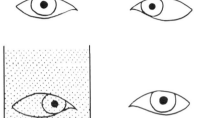

Fixating eye covered

Other eye moves to take up fixation

Cover/uncover test.

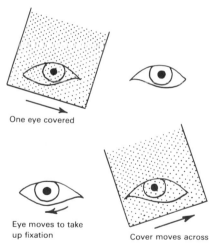

One eye covered

Eye moves to take up fixation

Cover moves across

Alternate cover test.

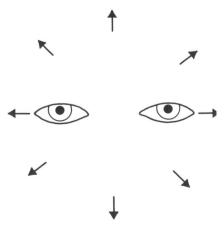

Test eye movements in all directions.

Adults may complain of deviation of the eyes or of diplopia. Children present because their parents or relatives notice the eye or eyes turning in or out, or there may be a family history of squint. Children may also be referred from vision screening clinics.

History

A family history of squint is a strong risk factor in the development of squint, and if there is any doubt the child should be referred. Children with disorders of the central nervous system such as cerebral palsy have a higher incidence of squint than normal children. Problems during birth and retarded development also increase the likelihood of a squint. The parents' visual problems should be ascertained, particularly large refractive errors.

The earlier the age of onset the more likely is the need for an operation. A constant squint has a worse visual prognosis than one that is intermittent.

Examination

● *Check the visual acuity*—If it does not correct with spectacles or a pinhole, ocular disease or amblyopia must be suspected. This is particularly important in children as the amblyopia or ocular problem must be treated immediately if the sight is to be preserved. Visual acuity in infants is difficult to assess. A history from the mother is useful to find out whether the baby looks at her and at objects. If, however, only one eye is affected the visual problem may not be apparent. If the sight is poor in only one eye, covering the good eye may make the child try to push the cover away. In an older child small coloured sweets may be used to get a rough estimate of acuity. The older child may also be able to match letters.

● *Look at the position of the patient's eyes*—Large squints will be obvious. Wide epicanthic folds may give the impression of a squint (pseudosquint), but children with wide epicanthic folds may still have true squints.

● *Look at the corneal reflections* of a bright light held in front of the eyes. Note the position of the reflections; they should be symmetrical. This test gives a rough estimate of the angle of any deviation.

● *Cover test*—There are two types of cover test that help to reveal a squint, especially if it is small and the examiner is unsure about the position of the corneal reflections. In the cover/uncover test one eye is covered and the other is observed. If the uncovered eye moves to fix on the object there is a squint that is present all the time, a manifest squint. The test should then be carried out on the other eye. A problem arises when the vision in the squinting eye is reduced, and the eye may not be able to take up fixation. This emphasises the need to test the vision of any patient with a squint. If the cover/uncover test is normal (indicating no manifest squint) the alternate cover test should be done. In this test the occluder is moved to and fro between the eyes. If the eye that has been uncovered moves then there is a latent squint.

● *Test eye movements in all directions of gaze*—If there is a paralytic squint, the degree of deviation will vary with the direction of gaze. An adult will often say that the separation of the images varies, and increases in the direction of action of the weakened muscles.

Squint

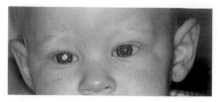

White reflex of retinoblastoma.

● *Examine the eye with a pupil dilating agent (mydriatic) and a ciliary muscle relaxing agent (cycloplegic)*—Any overt abnormalities of the eye should be noted. The reason for dilating the pupil is to exclude retinal disease such as retinoblastoma, and the cycloplegic allows a check for any refractive error. Adequate examination of the peripheral fundus and refraction require dilatation of the pupil and special equipment. Nevertheless, cataracts and other opacities in the media, and the white reflex that is suggestive of retinoblastoma, can often be detected by looking at the red reflex without dilating the pupil.

Management

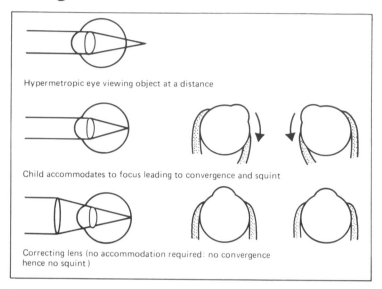

Hypermetropic eye viewing object at a distance

Child accommodates to focus leading to convergence and squint

Correcting lens (no accommodation required: no convergence hence no squint)

Spectacles to treat an accommodative convergent squint.

Paralytic squints usually occur in adults. Underlying conditions such as raised intracranial pressure, compressive lesions, and diseases such as diabetes, hypertension, myasthenia gravis and dysthyroid eye disease should be excluded. If diplopia is a problem one eye may need to be occluded temporarily—for example, by a patch stuck to the patients's spectacles. Alternatively, temporary prisms may be stuck on to the spectacles to eliminate the diplopia. Operation on the ocular muscles may be indicated if the squint stabilises. If an operation on the muscles either is not appropriate or proves inadequate permanent prisms may be incorporated into the spectacle prescription. Occasionally injection of minute doses of botulinum toxin into overacting muscles may reduce symptoms temporarily.

Non-paralytic squints usually occur in children. If the squint is caused by disease in the eye that is itself causing reduced vision and subsequent deviation of the eye—for example, cataract—this needs to be treated. Types of treatment for non-paralytic squints are listed below.

● *Spectacles*—There are two main indications for prescribing spectacles. Firstly, they should be given to the child who is hypermetropic (longsighted) and has a convergent squint. Normally when the ciliary muscle contracts the lens becomes more globular to allow the eye to focus on close objects (accommodation). This is linked to convergence so that both eyes can fix on the close object. If the child is hypermetropic the ciliary muscle has to contract strongly for the child to be able to focus on a near object. This excessive accommodation may cause overconvergence so that a squint occurs. This is termed an accommodative convergent squint. The use of hypermetropic glasses in this case relaxes the ciliary muscles and removes the drive to overconverge. Occasionally long acting drops that contract the ciliary muscle (such as ecothiopate iodide) may be used. These may, however, cause iris cysts and they should always be stopped before a general anaesthetic as they may impair recovery from muscle relaxants.

Secondly, spectacles are prescribed for the child who has a refractive error, particularly if this is unilateral. As a consequence of the refractive error the image on the retina will be indistinct. The visual

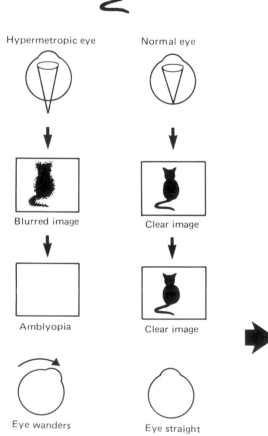

Hypermetropic eye   Normal eye

Blurred image   Clear image

Amblyopia   Clear image

Eye wanders   Eye straight

Amblyopia and squint caused by refractive error.

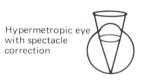

Hypermetropic eye with spectacle correction

Normal eye

No amblyopia No squint

Clear image   Clear image

Spectacles to treat refractive error and prevent amblyopia and squint.

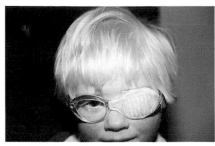

Good eye being occluded to stimulate amblyopic eye.

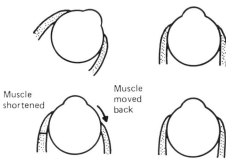

Muscle shortened

Muscle moved back

Operation for squint.

pathways will then not develop properly (resulting in amblyopia). Such children may not develop a squint until the vision is poor in one eye. This point emphasises the need to check the visual acuity. The use of glasses may therefore prevent severe visual loss in an otherwise "normal" eye—hence the need to refract every child with a squint or impaired vision.

● *Occlusion*—This is the familiar patching of one eye to encourage the development of the visual pathway of the "bad" eye. If the development of one pathway has been retarded by a squint or a refractive error this pathway can be stimulated if the "good" eye is patched. This can, however, be done for only a limited period, and there is a danger of the good eye itself becoming amblyopic. The underlying problem must, of course, be corrected in the meantime. The vision of the good eye may also be "blurred" with drops such as atropine.

● *Orthoptic treatment*—A series of visual exercises may encourage the simultaneous use of both eyes.

● *Operation*–The ocular muscles can be repositioned to straighten the eyes. Spectacles are prescribed and occlusion performed before operation because an eye is more likely to stay straight if the vision is good.

The effectiveness of treatment in reversing amblyopia decreases as the child gets older. Once the child is about 8 or 9 years old the visual system is no longer flexible and amblyopia cannot be reversed. The child may, however, still need glasses to correct refractive errors, and an operation may be required if there is a cosmetic problem.

GENERAL MEDICAL DISORDERS AND THE EYE

- Diabetes mellitus
- Hypertension
- Dysthyroid eye disease
- Rheumatoid arthritis
- Other arthritides
- Rosacea
- Sarcoid
- Congenital rubella
- AIDS

There are few serious medical conditions that do not affect the eye. It is important to know the ocular manifestations of systemic diseases for a variety of reasons.

- *Screening is required to detect early ocular changes that may require treatment to prevent blindness.* A good example is a diabetic with new vessels on the optic disc, which signal an exceptionally high risk of visual loss unless treatment is given in time.
- *Knowledge of the ocular complications of other diseases may help in the diagnosis of an ocular problem.* A red, locally injected, and tender eye in a patient with rheumatoid arthritis suggests scleritis, which may progress to perforation of the eye. Iritis should be strongly considered in a young man with ankylosing spondylitis who presents with a red eye.
- *The ocular symptoms may suggest the systemic disease*—for example, prominent eyes and lid lag in hyperthyroidism—*or confirm it*—for example, the Kayser-Fleisher ring of copper in Wilson's disease.
- *The ocular signs may have prognostic value.* If cotton wool spots occur in the eyes of a patient with otherwise asymptomatic AIDS the prognosis is particularly poor.

Diabetes mellitus

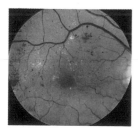

Background retinopathy: hard exudates, microaneurysms, and haemorrhages.

Diabetes mellitus is the commonest cause of blindness among people of working age in the Western world. Two per cent of the diabetic population are blind, many of them in the younger age groups. Much of this eye disease can now be prevented by treatment, which makes early identification and referral crucial. This section will concentrate on the treatable causes of visual loss in diabetics, and how they can be detected early enough to be treated effectively.

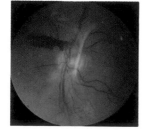

Proliferative retinopathy: new vessels, fibrosis, and haemorrhage.

Cataract and primary open angle glaucoma are more common in diabetic than in non-diabetic patients. Cataract can be treated by surgical removal, and primary open angle glaucoma may be treated by drugs and operations that lower the intraocular pressure. They can often be detected by viewing the red reflex and examining the optic disc, respectively. It is only too easy to forget to look for glaucomatous cupping of the disc when looking for the signs of diabetic retinopathy.

Cataract in a diabetic patient.

Blinding diabetic retinopathy occurs in both insulin-dependent and non-insulin-dependent diabetics and affects all age groups. The longer the duration of the diabetes, the more likely the patient is to have retinopathy (about 80% are affected after 20 years). Again this applies to all categories of diabetics. Diabetics should have their pupils dilated yearly with tropicamide 1% and the fundi examined if important physical signs are not to be missed. There are two main clinical types of retinopathy that cause blindness in diabetics, and these need to be identified and the patients referred for early treatment.

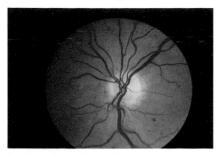

Background retinopathy with good acuity: regular review.

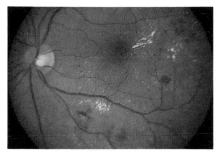

Background retinopathy with macular changes and good vision: refer.

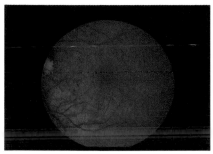

Background retinopathy with impaired acuity: refer.

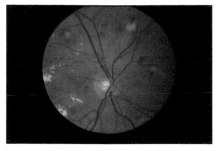

Preproliferative retinopathy. Cotton wool spots, large haemorrhages, and tortuous veins: refer urgently.

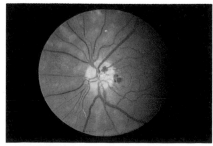

Proliferative retinopathy: refer immediately.

Background retinopathy is typified by microaneurysms, dot haemorrhages, and hard yellow exudates with well defined edges. These changes do not have much effect on vision when they occur in the peripheral retina. When they occur in the macular area, however, central vision may be severely affected. Background retinopathy at the macula (diabetic maculopathy) is the major cause of blindness in maturity onset diabetes, but it also occurs in younger, insulin-dependent diabetics. It may be amenable to focal laser photocoagulation, which may help to reduce any leakage. This is particularly true when hard exudates are a prominent feature of the maculopathy.

Proliferative retinopathy is typified by the growth of new vessels on the retina or into the vitreous cavity. This is thought to be due to the ischaemic diabetic retina producing vasoproliferative factors that cause the growth of abnormal new vessels. These vessels may bleed causing a sudden decrease in vision due to a vitreous haemorrhage. Worst still, this blood often results in the production of contractile membranes that gradually pull off the retina, causing blindness. This may occur in any diabetic, but more commonly in young, insulin-dependent patients. The vision may be 6/6 right up to the moment of a bleed, hence the need for early detection of new vessels by adequate fundal examination. New vessels may also grow on to the iris and occlude the drainage angle of the anterior chamber causing a painful hard eye (rubeotic glaucoma).

Laser (or any other method of photocoagulation) is also used to treat proliferative retinopathy. The laser, however, is not usually used directly to coagulate new vessels as these may bleed or recur. When a patient has new vessels at the disc the entire retina is treated with a laser, except for the macular area, which preserves the central vision. Hence the term "panretinal photocoagulation" or "pattern bombing". This destroys much of the ischaemic peripheral retina and stops it producing the vasoproliferative factors that induce the growth of new vessels, and often the new vessels regress. New blood vessels on the iris that block the outflow of aqueous and cause rubeotic glaucoma may also regress. It may, however, require thousands of laser burns and repeated treatments to achieve this. This treatment may significantly reduce peripheral vision and mean that the patient may have to give up driving.

Screening

Patients may be divided into the following groups for screening purposes.

(1) Those with no retinopathy or with background retinopathy and normal vision when tested with glasses or pinhole. These patients can be reviewed yearly with dilatation of the pupils. They should be told to attend sooner if there is a change in vision that is not corrected with glasses.

(2) Those with background retinopathy and changes around the macular area. They should be referred to an ophthalmologist as this may herald a blinding maculopathy.

(3) Those with background retinopathy and impaired acuity not corrected with glasses or pinhole. It may be that the patient has an oedematous or ischaemic form of maculopathy that is extremely hard to diagnose with the direct ophthalmoscope alone. The oedematous form may respond to focal laser treatment if this is given early.

(4) Those with preproliferative retinopathy. They have no new vessels, but the haemorrhages are larger, the veins are tortuous, and there are cotton wool spots. These physical signs imply that the retina is ischaemic and that there is a high risk that new vessels will subsequently form. These patients should be referred urgently.

(5) Those with proliferative retinopathy. This is typified by new blood vessels, and sometimes soft cotton wool spots, fibrosis, and vitreous haemorrhages. These patients need immediate referral, particularly if there are vitreous haemorrhages.

In addition to ocular treatment, blood sugar concentrations should be carefully controlled. If the blood sugar concentration is brought under control rapidly the fundus should be reviewed regularly during this period as there may be a transient worsening of the retinopathy.

- Control blood sugar
- Control hypertension
- Control hyperlipidaemia
- **Stop smoking**

Hypertension and hyperlipidaemia worsen the prognosis of retinopathy and must also be controlled. Patients should be told that it is essential to stop smoking.

Diabetics are also more prone to recurrent corneal abrasions, retinal vein occlusions, and cranial nerve palsies. Aids for a diabetic with impaired vision include an audible click count syringe, and a Hypotest instrument that gives an audible signal with urinary Diastix.

Hypertension

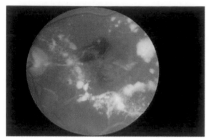

Retinopathy in malignant hypertension with macular exudates and occluded vessels; disc swelling has resolved.

The mild fundal changes of hypertension are extremely common. "Silver wiring" of the retinal arteries and arteriovenous nipping are well known signs, but arteriolar narrowing is the most reliable fundal sign.

Malignant hypertension is classically associated with swelling of the head of the optic nerve. Any patient with hard exudates, cotton wool spots, or haemorrhages due to hypertension has a grave prognosis. Patients with these fundal signs should have their blood pressure checked and diabetes excluded. Urgent referral to a physician is required, as this combination of signs is associated with life threatening hypertensive disease, and it may also result in blindness. Retinal vein occlusion is also more common in hypertensive patients.

Dysthyroid eye disease

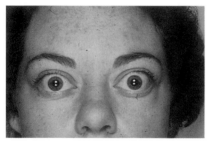

Hyperthyroidism with lid retraction.

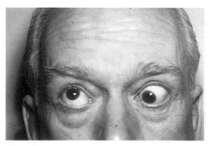

Autoimmune eye disease with restriction of ocular movements.

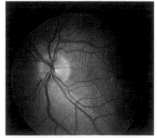

Choroidal folds.

Patients may have signs associated with hyperthyroidism and the consequent overactivity of the sympathetic system. These patients have retracted upper and lower lids caused by excessive stimulation of the sympathetically innervated muscles in the eyelids. This also gives rise to the well known sign of lid lag when the patient looks downwards. These features may suggest the diagnosis when the patient walks into the surgery.

If these signs are present thyroid dysfunction should be excluded. If there are no visual problems, no corneal exposure, and the eyes move normally the patient need not be referred. Patients may, however, also have evidence of autoimmune disease directed against the orbital contents, particularly the muscles. These signs may be associated with the classic signs of Graves' disease including goitre, pseudoclubbing of the fingers (thyroid acropathy), hyperthyroidism, and pretibial myxoedema. Autoimmune ocular disease may also occur on its own with no thyroid dysfunction. The clinical features include:

- *Swelling of the eyelids.*
- *Oedema (chemosis) and injection of the conjunctiva.*
- *Exposure of the cornea* because of lack of blinking and failure of the lids to cover the eye adequately.
- *Pronounced protrusion of the eyes.* The absence of this feature in association with the other features may be even more serious as it may be that a tight orbital septal wall is holding back the swollen orbital contents. This may lead to a rise in intraocular pressure as well as pressure on the optic nerve.
- *Restriction of eye movements.* This is caused by infiltration of the muscles with inflammatory cells and consequent inflammation, oedema, and finally fibrosis.
- *Optic neuropathy.* This is comparatively rare, but the fundal signs include vascular congestion and swelling or atrophy of the head of the optic nerve. There may be "folds" in the choroid caused by pressure on the globe. Optic neuropathy should be excluded in any patient with autoimmune eye disease who experiences visual deterioration.
- These features may occur in any combination.

Management

- Associated thyroid dysfunction should be excluded, though treatment of any dysfunction may make no difference to the eye disease and may even make it worse.
- Artificial tears should be used to lubricate the cornea and prevent drying and corneal ulceration.

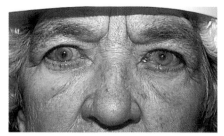

Patient with mild dysthyroid eye disease. Red eyes and exposure due to infrequent blinking.

- If there are cosmetic or exposure problems caused by lid retraction guanethidine drops 5% may reduce the lid retraction by relaxing the sympathetically controlled retractor muscles. Occasionally an operation on these muscles and associated lid structures may be required to reverse the lid retraction.
- If corneal exposure is threatening sight the eyelids may have to be sewn together temporarily (tarsorrhaphy).
- Prisms incorporated in the patient's glasses may help to correct any double vision.
- Operations on the muscles of eye movement may be required to realign the eyes in patients with longstanding diplopia that has stabilised. Recently the introduction of local injections of minute doses of botulinum toxin to paralyse specific extraocular muscles has meant that patients with restrictive muscle diseases may sometimes be treated at an earlier stage.
- In serious disease with corneal problems or pressure on the optic nerve emergency treatment may be required, which may include high doses of steroids, surgical orbital decompression, and radiotherapy. The visual fields may be restricted and there may be a relative afferent pupillary defect. Changes in colour vision, which may sometimes be noticed while watching colour television, may be an important sign of optic nerve compression and patients should be told to inform the doctor immediately if these changes are noticed.

- Protect cornea
- Prevent damage to optic nerve

Rheumatoid arthritis

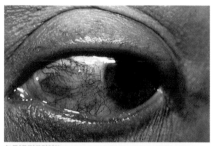

Episcleritis.

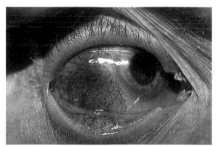

Scleritis.

Rheumatoid arthritis is another common disease in which ocular complications are frequent. The lacrimal glands are also affected by an inflammatory process with consequent inadequate tear flow. The patient complains of dry, gritty, and sore eyes. Treatment consists of replacement artificial tear drops instilled as often as necessary. Simple ointment may also help, but this will blur the vision if used during the day. If there is an aggregation of mucus, mucolytic eye drops—for example, acetylcysteine—may help, but patients should be warned that these sting.

The inflammatory process may also affect the episcleral and scleral coats of the eye causing the patient to complain of a red, uncomfortable eye. The redness is usually focal and there is tenderness over the area. Scleritis is usually much more painful than episcleritis and the injected vessels are deeper. If scleritis continues the sclera may become thin (scleromalacia) and the eye may eventually perforate (scleromalacia perforans). The patient should be referred, as systemic treatment may be indicated.

These processes may also occur in other connective tissue diseases such as systemic lupus erythematosus, scleroderma, and dermatomyositis.

Other arthritides

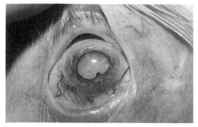

Chronic anterior uveitis and secondary cataract in seronegative arthritis.

The seronegative arthritides include ankylosing spondylitis, Reiter's syndrome, psoriatic arthritis, and arthritis associated with inflammatory bowel disease. Acute anterior uveitis (iritis, iridocyclitis) is much more common in these patients. If a patient with any of these conditions has a red eye anterior uveitis should be suspected. This is particularly true if the patient has had past attacks, and "experienced" patients often know when an attack is coming on. The patient should be referred for early treatment, which may prevent some of the complications of anterior uveitis.

Seronegative childhood arthritis is a particularly important cause of chronic anterior uveitis. The great danger is that the eyes in this condition are often white and pain free and the child may not complain of any visual problems. There may also be secondary cataracts that may cause irreversible amblyopia. Glaucoma secondary to the anterior uveitis may also occur, and may be asymptomatic until the vision has been

Risk factors for ocular involvement in childhood seronegative arthritis

* Female
* <5 joints affected
* Antinuclear antibodies

severely damaged. The groups of children particularly at risk are females, those with fewer than five joints affected by the arthritis (pauciarticular), and those with antinuclear antibodies in their blood. These children should be referred to an ophthalmologist.

Rosacea

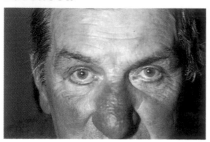

Acne rosacea and associated blepharitis.

Rosacea may seriously affect the eyes. There is often associated blepharitis, which may result in recurrent chalazia and styes. The abnormal lids and lipid secretion affect the tear film and the symptoms of "dry eye" result. The cornea scars, particularly in the inferonasal and inferotemporal areas, with corneal neovascularisation. Thinning occurs and the cornea may occasionally perforate.

Treatment with tear substitutes is indicated with treatment for any associated blepharitis. Systemic tetracycline (250 mg four times daily for up to a month, then daily for several months) may considerably improve the patient's ocular as well as facial condition.

Sarcoid

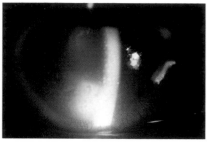

Anterior uveitis in sarcoidosis: large deposits of inflammatory white cells on posterior surface of cornea.

Sarcoid is associated with various ocular problems. Acute uveitis and chronic uveitis occur, which may result in cataract, glaucoma, and a band of calcium deposited in the cornea (band keratopathy). The lacrimal glands may be infiltrated resulting in symptoms of "dry eye" requiring tear replacement. The granulomatous process may also affect the posterior part of the eye in the form of vasculitis and sometimes infiltration of the optic nerve.

Congenital rubella

* Cataract
* Squint
* Refractive error
* Glaucoma
* Retinopathy

The ocular manifestations of congenital rubella are extremely important. The child may be mentally retarded and deaf, thus early recognition of ocular problems and their treatment are vital. The treatable defects include cataract, glaucoma, squint, and refractive errors. The cataract may not appear until several weeks or months after birth, so the eyes should be re-examined. There may be a diffuse retinopathy ("salt and pepper" appearance).

Acquired immune deficiency syndrome (AIDS)

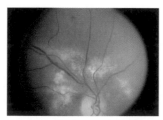

Cytomegalovirus retinitis in AIDS.

The ocular complications of AIDS may be blinding. Manifestations include Kaposi's sarcoma of the conjunctiva, retinal haemorrhages, and vasculitis. Cotton wool spots may appear and disappear spontaneously, and their presence signifies a poor prognosis even in a patient without symptoms. Ocular cytomegalovirus infection presents as areas of opacification with haemorrhages and exudates that proceed to severe ocular damage, including retinal detachment. Various antiviral agents, however, have proved useful in the treatment of ocular complications, but they may have to be taken continuously and systemic side effects are common. Blindness as a result of the ocular complications of AIDS is one of the main reasons for suicide in patients with AIDS.

THE EYE AND THE NERVOUS SYSTEM

Nerves of eye movement

Ocular signs may be the first indication of serious neurological disease. Alternatively, the eyes may be responsible for "neurological" symptoms such as headache.

Palsies of the third, fourth, and sixth cranial nerves all cause paralytic squints in which the angle of the squint varies with the direction of the gaze. Adult patients may also complain of double vision, so it is important to exclude palsies of these three nerves when examining patients who have either a squint or double vision.

Third nerve palsy—A patient with a third nerve palsy may present with a variety of symptoms depending on the cause of the palsy. He may complain of a drooping eyelid, double vision (if the lid does not cover the eye), or headache in the distribution of the ophthalmic division of the trigeminal nerve. On examination there is characteristically a ptosis (drooping eyelid) due to a paralysed levator muscle of the eyelid and the eye is turned out because of the action of the unaffected lateral rectus muscle that is supplied by the sixth nerve. The eye is sometimes turned slightly downwards due to the unopposed action of the unaffected superior oblique muscle supplied by the fourth nerve. The pupil is dilated because the parasympathetic fibres of the third nerve supplying the sphincter pupillae are damaged. Important causes of a third nerve palsy include intracranial aneurysms, compressive lesions in the cavernous sinus, and diabetes. The presence of pain and a dilated pupil mean that a compressive lesion must be excluded urgently, as treatment may be life saving and curative for what may be an otherwise fatal lesion such as an aneurysm.

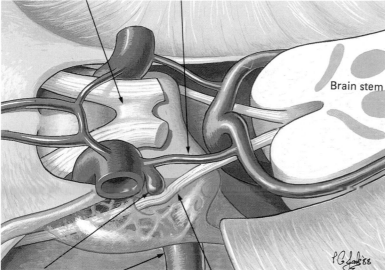

Optic chiasm   Posterior communicating artery

Brain stem

Aneurysm   Internal carotid artery   Third nerve

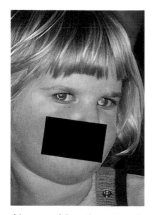

Abnormal head posture in right fourth nerve palsy.

Fourth nerve palsy—This is often difficult to diagnose. There may be a compensatory head tilt in that the head will be tilted away from the side of the lesion and the chin will be depressed. The fourth nerve is long and is therefore particularly susceptible to injury. A patient with bilateral fourth nerve palsies due to a head injury may complain only of difficulty in reading. This is due to difficulty during depression and convergence of the eyes because both superior oblique muscles are paralysed. This diagnosis should be considered in any patient who complains of difficulty in reading after a head injury.

Sixth nerve palsy—This is probably the best known of the palsies of the three nerves of ocular motility. The eye on the affected side cannot be abducted. The patient develops horizontal diplopia that worsens when he looks towards the side of the affected muscle. It is important to recognise a sixth nerve palsy as it may be due to raised intracranial pressure that is causing compression of the sixth nerve.

Management—This is initially directed to making an accurate diagnosis. If diplopia is a problem, sticky tape may be placed over the patient's glasses, or a patch may be put over the eye. Adults will not develop amblyopia. Temporary prisms may be placed over the glasses if the angle of deviation is not too large. For long term treatment, permanent prisms (which are clearer than temporary prisms) may be incorporated into a prescription for spectacles. Later, an operation may be performed to straighten the eyes.

- **Diagnosis**
- Patch
- Temporary prism
- Permanent prism
- ? Operation

Facial nerve palsy

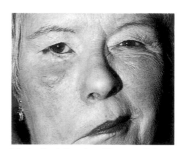

Right facial palsy. The eyelids on the right have been partly sewn together to protect the eye.

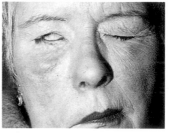

Cornea moves up under upper lid on attempted closure of the eyelid.

Seventh nerve palsy

Facial weakness due to a seventh nerve palsy is common. In many cases no cause is found and the palsy improves spontaneously. If the eyelids do not close properly corneal exposure, ulceration, and eventual scarring and blindness may result. Ocular assessment should include:
- *Testing of corneal sensation*—The cornea is innervated by the ophthalmic branch of the fifth nerve. If the corneal sensation is impaired the patient should be referred to an ophthalmic surgeon, as there is a high risk of corneal scarring. Patients cannot feel foreign bodies or feel when their corneas are ulcerating. This is in addition to being unable to close the eye and lubricate the cornea.
- *Testing of Bell's phenomenon* (not to be confused with Bell's palsy)—Normally when the eyes are closed they move up under the upper lid. This "Bell's phenomenon" may be tested by asking the patient with a facial palsy to close his eyes while the observer watches the position of the cornea. If the cornea does not move up under the paralysed lid the patient is at high risk of developing corneal exposure.
- *Staining the cornea with fluorescein*—If there is staining of the cornea when fluorescein is used this indicates that the cornea is drying out. If there is only a tiny amount of stain, the eye is white and quiet, and the visual acuity is normal the patient may be managed in the short term with tear drops and ointment. If the staining persists or if the eye becomes red then he should be referred straight away. The cornea may need to be protected by frequent lubrication and possibly sewing together the lateral parts of the eyelids or lowering the upper eyelid with botulinum toxin.

Sympathetic pathway

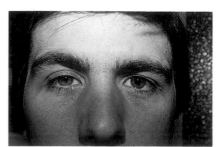

Right Horner's syndrome.

Horner's syndrome

In a patient with Horner's syndrome the sympathetic nerve supply to the eye is disturbed. The clinical features are:
- *A small pupil that is reactive to light* (unlike the small pupil due to pilocarpine eye drops) because only the sympathetically innervated dilator muscle of the pupil is paralysed and not the parasympathetically innervated constrictor muscle.
- *A drooping eyelid*—The muscles that raise the eyelid are innervated by the third nerve and also by the sympathetic nerve supply. Thus lesions of either the third nerve or the sympathetic nervous system supplying these muscles cause a ptosis, though in the latter case it is only slight.

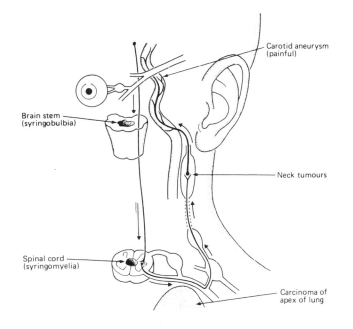

Carotid aneurysm (painful)

Brain stem (syringobulbia)

Neck tumours

Spinal cord (syringomyelia)

Carcinoma of apex of lung

Sites of lesions of the sympathetic pathway to the eye.

• *Lack of sweating on the same side of the face* is again because of sympathetic denervation and depends on the position of the lesion. The ocular movements are completely normal as the muscles of the globe are not sympathetically innervated. The figure shows the pathways of the sympathetic system and possible causes of Horner's syndrome.

Optic disc

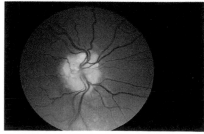

Swollen disc caused by raised intracranial pressure (papilloedema).

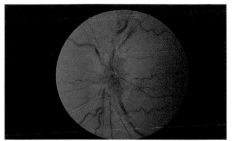

Swollen disc caused by giant cell arteritis.

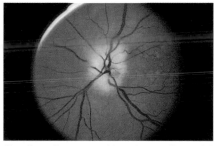

Swollen disc caused by retinal vein occlusion.

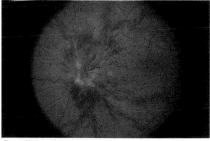

Drusen.

The swollen optic disc

There are many causes of a swollen optic disc, the best known of which is raised intracranial pressure resulting in the development of papilloedema. *The absence of papilloedema, however, does not exclude raised intracranial pressure.* It is the history and examination of the patient that should lead to the suspicion of raised intracranial pressure, and a swollen optic disc is merely a helpful sign. The vision of patients with papilloedema is usually not affected until late in the course of the disease. Most causes of a swollen disc are serious from either the ocular or the systemic point of view, and patients should be referred promptly. If a patient has a swollen optic disc the following features suggest a diagnosis other than raised intracranial pressure.

• *Impaired vision*—Vision is usually impaired only late in the course of papilloedema. It is crucial to consider giant cell arteritis in the presence of impaired vision and the patient may or may not have, in addition, aching muscles, malaise, headaches, tenderness over the temporal arteries, and claudication of the jaw muscles when eating. The disc is characteristically swollen and pale because the small vessels that supply the head of the optic nerve are inflamed and occluded. By this time the vision will be severely affected. It is important to exclude giant cell arteritis in any patient over 60 with visual disturbance or a swollen optic disc as urgent treatment with steroids should be instituted to prevent blindness in the other eye.

• *Disturbance of the visual fields*—The visual fields of a patient with raised intracranial pressure are usually normal. The presence of a field defect should lead one to suspect some other diagnosis such as compression of the optic nerve.

• *A pale disc*—The disc of a patient with raised intracranial pressure is often hyperaemic. It is only in longstanding papilloedema that the discs become atrophic and pale. The disc is also pale if the swelling is due to ischaemia of the optic nerve as in giant cell arteritis.

• *Retinal exudates and haemorrhages*—These are present in papilloedema and are usually around the disc. If there are many exudates or haemorrhages in the retina diagnoses such as retinal vein occlusion, malignant hypertension, diabetes, and vasculitis should be considered. In all patients the blood pressure should be measured and the urine tested for the presence of sugar, blood, and protein.

Conditions that may mimic swelling of the head of the optic nerve include:

• *Long sightedness* (hypermetropia), in which the margin of the optic disc does not look clear. A clue lies in the patient's glasses; hypermetropic correcting lenses make the eyes look larger.

The eye and the nervous system

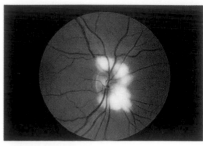

Myelinated nerve fibres.

- *Drusen of the head of the optic nerve*—These colloid bodies of the head of the nerve make the margin of the disc look blurred.
- *Developmental abnormalities of the head of the nerve*—These, however, may be difficult to diagnose.

Pale optic disc

There are many causes of a pale optic disc and it is important to make the correct diagnosis as many of them are treatable. These include compressive lesions, glaucoma, vitamin deficiency, the presence of toxic substances—for example, lead or some drugs—and infective conditions such as syphilis. It is also important to identify whether the cause is hereditary as genetic counselling and, occasionally, metabolic treatments are available—for example, a diet free of phytanic acid and plasma exchange may prevent the progression of ocular disease in Refsum's disease.

Headaches and the eye

Important features

- Nature of pain
- Associated visual disturbance
- Red eye
- Defective ocular movements
- Abnormal pupils
- Abnormal optic disc

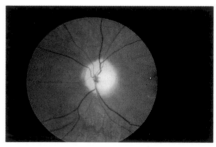

Optic atrophy.

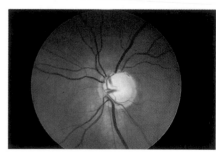

Glaucomatous cupping.

Most patients who present with a history of "headache" around the eye do not have serious disease. Points in the history and examination that should raise suspicion of serious disease include:

The nature of the headache—Headaches that cause sleep disturbance, or that are worse on waking or with coughing, suggest raised intracranial pressure. Temporal tenderness in patients over the age of 60 with symptoms of aching muscles and malaise suggest giant cell arteritis.

Visual disturbance—If there is a change in visual acuity that cannot be corrected by a pinhole test, serious disease should be suspected. A history of haloes around lights (due to transient oedema of the cornea when the intraocular pressure rises with the headache) suggests attacks of angle closure glaucoma.

A red eye—In acute glaucoma the eye is usually red, injected, and tender, and the acuity is diminished. The pain is deep seated and may be associated with vomiting. Inflammation of the iris and ciliary body also cause a red eye and a deep pain. Primary open angle glaucoma does not present with severe pain.

Defective ocular movements—If there are restricted ocular movements on the same side as the pain serious disease must be suspected. This may include orbital cellulitis (from infected sinuses), inflammatory lesions in the orbit, and compressive lesions causing nerve palsies—for example, a posterior communicating aneurysm causing a third nerve palsy and pain around the eye.

Abnormal pupils—An abnormal pupil on the side of the headache should suggest a compressive lesion—for example, a painful Horner's syndrome due to an internal carotid aneurysm.

In so called "cluster headaches" and "ophthalmoplegic migraine" pupillary abnormalities and ocular motility problems may be present in these relatively benign conditions. Patients with headache around the eye, however, together with ocular motility or pupillary abnormalities, should be investigated to exclude serious lesions.

Swelling, atrophy, or cupping of the optic disc—If a patient with headaches around the eye has any of these findings referral is required. The swelling and atrophy may be due to a compressive lesion and pathological cupping suggests a chronic form of glaucoma.

INDEX

Index